Praise for Ian

She Com

"Every man's must-read. Tell your guy to put down the remote and pick up *She Comes First*." —*Cosmopolitan*

"Is it too late to nominate Kerner for some sort of Nobel prize?" —*Blogcritics*

"Kerner has devoted his life to the study and practice of good sex—there are few men that wouldn't benefit from the female-centric philosophy and techniques that Kerner advocates." —*Salon*

"*She Comes First* is quite simply the best guide to oral sex out there." —AskMen.com

"The man who made oral sex into an art form." —Pepper Schwartz, Ph.D., Professor of Sociology, University of Washington, and author of *Prime: Adventures and Advice on Sex, Love, and the Sensual Years*

"Women will be putty in your hands if you read this book!" —Anka Radakovich, author of *The Wild Girls Club*

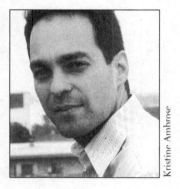

Kristine Ambrose

About the Author

IAN is a sex therapist and *New York Times* bestselling author of numerous books on the subject. He was born and raised in New York City, where he resides with his wife and two sons.

SHE COMES FIRST

Ian Kerner, Ph.D.

SHE

The Thinking Man's Guide

COMES

to Pleasuring a Woman

FIRST

WILLIAM MORROW
An Imprint of HarperCollins*Publishers*

A hardcover edition of this book was published in 2004
by ReganBooks, an imprint of HarperCollins Publishers.

HarperCollins books may be purchased for educational,
business, or sales promotional use. For information, please e-mail
the Special Markets Department at SPsales@harpercollins.com.

FIRST HARPER PAPERBACK PUBLISHED 2010.

Designed by Kate Nichols

Illustrations by Naomi Pitcairn

The Library of Congress has catalogued the hardcover edition as follows:

Kerner, Ian.
    She comes first : the thinking man's guide to pleasuring a woman / Ian Kerner.—
1st ed.
        p. cm.
    Includes bibliographical references.
    ISBN 0-06-053825-2
    1. Sex instruction for men.   2. Oral sex.   3. Female orgasm.   I. Title.
HQ36.K47 2004
                                                                          2004041787

    ISBN 978-0-06-053826-2 (pbk.)

23 24 25 26 27 LBC 34 33 32 31 30

For my wife, Lisa

*"You should be kissed, and often, and by
someone who knows how."*

—Clark Gable,
Gone with the Wind

Contents

Part Two: Rules of Usage

Part Three: Putting It All Together

SHE COMES FIRST

Introduction: Confessions of a Premature Ejaculator

THE PREMISE of this book is simple: when it comes to pleasuring women and conversing in the language of love, cunnilingus should be every man's native tongue. As bestselling sex author Lou Paget has written, "Ask most women, and if they're being honest, they will admit that what makes them hottest and come hardest is when a man can use his tongue well."

But as with any language, in order to express yourself fluently, in order to make your subject sing and soar, you must be thoroughly acquainted with the rules of grammar and style. One of my favorite books on the subject is the indispensable classic *Elements of Style*. I don't think I would have made it through freshman comp, or survived college as an English major, without that slim, dog-eared paperback tucked away in my back pocket. In the able hands of authors Strunk and White, grammar was not simply made understandable and meaningful—it was made beautiful.

Elements of Style exhorted readers to "write boldly and make definite assertions." And in the spirit of that timeless classic, *She Comes First* will condense a wealth of experience and expertise into a simple, essential rule book; it will elaborate on the principles and philosophy that underlie those rules and, in doing so, offer nothing less than the definitive guide to the grammar of oral sex. If you want to learn how to give a woman mind-blowing, body-rippling orgasms with your tongue *every* time, this is the book for you.

Although I am a sex therapist, this book is also written from a practitioner's perspective; by someone who knows and loves cunnilingus, appreciates its role in stimulating female sexual response, and has developed a methodology for consistently leading women to orgasm: one that stems from the conviction that cunnilingus is much more than just a sexual activity, but rather the centerpiece of a philosophy of sexual contentment. Call it the "way of the tongue."

But don't get me wrong: I'm not some Casanova or Don Juan, vainly putting words down on paper in order to boast and strut—far from it. Through much of my life I've suffered terribly from sexual dysfunction, and I know all too well the humiliation, anxiety, and despair of not being able to satisfy a woman. If anything, this book was written in the sincere hope that other men might develop effective "sexual habits"—ones that will enable them, along with their partners, to suffer less than I have, or perhaps not at all.

My initial forays into oral sex were a way of compensating for my sexual inadequacies, and they were approached with the assumption that cunnilingus was a poor man's second to the joys and splendors of "real sex"—like many, I took it for granted that intercourse was the "right way" for couples to experience orgasms. But, to my surprise, I discovered that the "way of the tongue" was by no means inferior to intercourse; if anything, it was superior, in many cases the only way in which women were able to receive the persistent, rhythmic stimulation, outside of masturbation, necessary to achieve an orgasm. I quickly learned that oral sex *is* real sex, and later in life, when I happened to come across a copy of the seminal *Hite Report on Female Sexuality*, I was reassured to find that women consider oral sex to be "one of their most favorite and exciting activities; women mentioned over and over how much they loved it." When it comes to pleasure, there is no right or wrong way to have an orgasm—the only thing that's wrong is to assume that women need or value them any less than men do.

In her article "Just Be a Man: Six Simple Suggestions," sex columnist Amy Sohn's very first piece of advice is, "A man goes down. No excuses. No hesitation."

But once down there, what's a man to do? The vast majority of women complain about guys who don't like to do it, don't know how to do it, or simply don't do it nearly enough. Flannery O'Connor was right: a good man is hard to find, especially one who's good at taking a leisurely stroll downtown. But once found, a skilled cunnilinguist rarely goes unappreciated. In her essay "Lip Service: On Being a Cunning Linguist," author and sex columnist Anka Radakovich sings the praises of a boyfriend who specialized in oral sex: "I became tongue-whipped (the female equivalent of pussy-whipped) and even offered to do his laundry if he would come over and satisfy me. After two months, I put a framed photo of his tongue on my desk."

It's time to "think outside her box." When it comes to the oral caress, every man should make a mantra of Rhett Butler's infamous line to Scarlett O'Hara in *Gone with the Wind:* "You should be kissed, and often, and by someone who knows how."

Those who know me know I'm a private person. I wouldn't dream of confiding my battles with sexual dysfunction to the world if I didn't wholeheartedly believe that there was a compelling need for this book. I know this based on what I've read, what I've been told, and, most important, what I've experienced firsthand as a sex and relationships counselor: not only do most women crave and enjoy cunnilingus; they require it. Any sex therapist will tell you that the number one complaint they hear over and over from women is of an inability to experience orgasm during penis-vagina intercourse. The solution is not simply "more foreplay," as magazines often chide us, but rather the skillful extension of those activities we associate with foreplay, namely oral stimulation, into *complete*, fully realized acts of lovemaking—the transformation of foreplay into nothing less than *coreplay*.

This book is not anti-intercourse, but rather pro-"outercourse"—a conception of sex that goes beyond penetration, embraces *mutual* pleasure, and is better suited to stimulating the female sexual anatomy to orgasm. This model doesn't exclude intercourse, but instead promotes the postponement of male gratification until after a woman has achieved her *first* (but hopefully not last) orgasm during a session of sexual activity—a deferment that has the double benefit of vouchsafing female satisfaction while also significantly enhancing the quality of the male climax. This book espouses the postponement of gratification, *not* the postponement of enjoyment.

She Comes First offers men and women a "bird in the hand" approach to good sex, as opposed to the high-stakes "all or nothing" proposition of intercourse. It's time to close the sex gap and create a level playing field in the exchange of pleasure, and cunnilingus is far more than just a means for achieving this noble end; it's the cornerstone of a new sexual paradigm, one that exuberantly extols a *shared* experience of pleasure, intimacy, respect and contentment. It's also one of the greatest gifts of love a man can bestow upon a woman.

How to Read this Book

In Part I, The Elements of Sexual Style, you will be introduced to a powerful philosophy that will inform, if not dramatically alter, the way you approach sex and relationships. You will learn to:

- Dispense with "disinformation" and cultivate a true understanding of female sexuality

- Think *clitorally*, rather than *vaginally*; to focus on *stimulation* as opposed to *penetration*
- Postpone gratification without sacrificing pleasure
- Turn foreplay into coreplay
- Skillfully navigate the process of female sexual response and appreciate the role of the clitoris as the powerhouse of pleasure
- Develop a sense of awareness that will render the often elusive female orgasm knowable and tangible beyond the shadow of a doubt

We will also discuss important, often misunderstood, topics such as the "real" anatomy of the female genitalia, hygiene, safe sex, as well as the social and cultural context that informs the way we think and act regarding sex.

If Part I is the "why" of cunnilingus, then Part II, Rules of Usage, is the "how." Here you will be introduced to proven oral techniques that will enable you to successfully take a woman through the entire process of sexual response, or what I've dubbed the "play process"— foreplay, coreplay, and moreplay.

Whereas many sex books are content to merely tell the reader "what" to do, it's this author's conviction that the "when" is just as important. It's all in the timing, and to that end, Part III, Putting it Together, delineates clear routines for seamlessly integrating the techniques into a unified experience that will enable you and your partner to reach new erotic heights.

Peppered throughout the book you will also find illustrations, tips, exercises, interesting facts, frequently asked questions, as well as candid responses from some of the many men and women I interviewed regarding sex and relationships, as well as their own personal do's and don'ts.

Finally, at the end of the book you will find a series of appendices that address many relevant topics and specific situations.

Taken as a whole, *She Comes First* represents the most thorough treatment of the art of cunnilingus currently available, and will not only teach you everything you need to know in order to master the grammar of oral sex, but will also answer any questions you might have along the way.

By the time you finish this book, you'll not only be thinking about sex from a new perspective, but there will also be *nothing* you won't know about how to lead a woman to orgasm with your tongue time and time again.

Pop Quiz

Feel free to read *She Comes First* in whatever manner you find comfortable, but if you're inclined to skip Part I and go straight to the techniques in Part II, then I would ask you first to consider a few simple questions:

- Did you know that the clitoris has *eighteen* parts, all of which play a role in the production of pleasure? Can you identify them?
- Did you know that the vast majority of nerve endings that contribute to the female orgasm are concentrated on the surface of the vulva and do not require any penetration whatsoever in order to be stimulated to orgasm?
- Do you know the many different types of orgasms a woman is capable of experiencing?
- Can you say with complete confidence that you know how to locate the G-spot? Can you name any other hidden zones of pleasure?
- Do you know why cunnilingus is the best means of stimulating a woman to multiple orgasms?
- Do you know why a man is partially responsible for his partner's genital scent?

• Are you entirely sure that your partner has never faked an orgasm, and can you unequivocally recognize the difference between the real thing and a screaming phony?

If you answered no to any of these important questions, then I would encourage you to read the book from start to finish. But no matter how you choose to peruse *She Comes First*; I hope that, like *Elements of Style*, it proves to be a book you can come back to time and time again, regardless of your level of expertise.

A Taste of What's to Come

In the spirit of *Elements of Style*, here are a few basic rules to get you started:

1. Learn to Appreciate Irony: because when it comes to human sexuality, life abounds with it. Just for starters, take the fact that men and women's genitals are formed from the same embryonic tissue, yet our respective processes of arousal couldn't be more different. As the founding editors of *Men's Health* magazine, Stefan Bechtel and Laurence Roy Stains, so succinctly put it in their book *Sex: A Man's Guide*, "Studies show that three fourths of men are finished with sex within a few minutes of starting. But women often need 15 minutes or more to become sufficiently aroused for orgasm. And therein lies a world of rage, grief, and airborne pots and pans."

To put it in grammatical terms, most women are left frustrated with "incomplete sentences" in the face of their partners' prematurely "dangling participles." Hence this book's emphasis on the postponement of male gratification and the first part of its title: *She Comes First*. As journalist Paula Kamen documents in *Her Way, a Survey of Contemporary Young Women*, "Women's orgasms are no longer considered a lucky bonus or an afterthought, which marks a shift away from sexual guilt and toward women's pursuing their own desires, as men always have."

When it comes to pleasuring women, keep in mind the ancient words of Taoist master Wu Hsien, "The man must keep the situation in control and benefit from the communion without undue haste."

2. Don't Mistake Her Subject for an Object: namely, the clitoris. With its eight thousand nerve endings (twice as many as the penis), enviable ability to produce multiple orgasms during a single session of sex, and no known purpose other than pleasure, is it any wonder that sex therapists Masters and Johnson proclaimed the clitoris "a unique organ in the total of humanity"? The clitoris has over *eighteen* parts, both visible and hidden, that participate in the production of pleasure. (Keep reading, and you'll learn how to master each and every one of them.) Contrary to conventional wisdom—at least the kind that's as common as Ben-Gay and mildew in the men's locker room—the clitoris is much more than just a "love button," it's a sophisticated network of arousal that has more hot spots than a latent volcano.

3. The Tongue Is Mightier than the Sword: especially when it comes to clitoral stimulation. Even porn star Ron Jeremy, in possession of the famous ten-inch member, observed, "More women have gotten off with my tongue than with my penis." Shere Hite, author of the *Hite Report on Sexuality*, went so far as to suggest, "Intercourse was never meant to stimulate women to orgasm." One of the reasons for this is that the clitoris is about 2 to 3 cm closer to the front of the woman's body than the vaginal opening. During intercourse, the penis often misses the clitoris altogether.

In *Sex: A Man's Guide*, the authors cite a study in which ninety-eight wives in happy, stable marriages kept a sex diary that noted the frequency of sexual activity and the level of satisfaction. Of all the activities they mentioned, *cunnilingus ranked as the most satisfying.* Eighty-two percent said having their husbands pleasure them orally was very satisfying; the next highest activity, intercourse, was rated very satisfying by only 68 percent. The women reported that during intercourse they reached orgasm about 25 percent of the time. *But they reached orgasm 81 percent of the time during cral sex.* As Dr. Alex Comfort wrote of cunnilingus in *The New Joy of Sex,* "One can give the woman dozens of orgasms in this way and she may still want to go on from there."

4. Learn from Your Mistakes: Unlike the adolescent boys of the Cook Island of Mangaia, who are trained in the finer points of breast stimulation, cunnilingus, and delayed ejaculation in order to guarantee the pleasure of their future partners, our Western education is, alas, an incomplete one. When surveyed by Shere Hite regarding their partners' oral techniques, the vast majority of women complained that guys were too rough, too impatient; too fast, too slow; off target, or they changed rhythm at the wrong time. One woman even exclaimed, "It seems like he is trying to erase my clitoris."

Yikes!

But what many women don't know is that men yearn for feedback and guidance. They crave instruction, but communicating about sex is far from easy, and words often fail us in the heat of the moment. As author Sally Tisdale put it in her book *Talk Dirty to Me: An Intimate Philosophy of Sex,* "We can't really explain how arousal feels, what an orgasm is, and the closer we get to one, the less value words have, the less we can use language at all."

So we turn to sex books and magazines or, worse, cheesy porno flicks, and locker-room banter. Most books take an encyclopedic approach to sexuality—a little of everything, not a whole lot of anything. They emphasize breadth rather than depth and, *at best,* cunnilingus is given equal attention with other subjects. When it comes to detailing technique, most offer a few scanty pages at most, and almost all write about cunnilingus as an aspect of foreplay rather than as a complete process in its own right. They're like big fat cookbooks that are limited to a few recipes in each category. But cunnilingus is a repast in and of itself, and there are hundreds, if not thousands, of unique ways to partake.

Attention Men

While *She Comes First* will benefit anyone—straight or gay, male or female—who has an interest in learning about female orgasms and producing them consistently through inspired oral techniques, the book was written primarily for those guys of the world who crave the knowledge to become better, more sensitive lovers, and for the women in their lives who are eager to benefit from their education.

The truth is that men and women differ markedly in how they learn about sex. *The Kinsey Report*, a well-known survey of human sexuality, observed in 1953, "It is obvious that neither younger girls nor older women discuss their sexual experiences in the open in the ways that males do." A lot has changed since then. In an updated 1990 *Kinsey Report on Sexual Literacy*, the authors note that women aged eighteen to twenty-nine fared better than their male peers in terms of their knowledge of sexuality and attributed the differences to women's "growing belief that they have a right to sex information and accessible publications about women's health." So it would appear that both the women's movement and the safe-sex movement, with their emphases on clarity and candor, have done much to educate women about their bodies and sexuality in the last half century.

But what about guys?

In both my research and interviews I observed that the women were, in general, more knowledgeable about sex and tended to be much more willing to discuss sexual issues freely and candidly. In describing sexual activities, principally cunnilingus, women were significantly more aware of the qualitative aspects, as well as the technical details, related to their sexual response. While emphasizing the importance of personal experience in acquiring knowledge, women also confirmed that much of their information on sexuality came from friends and parents, as well as books, magazines, and the Internet.

Men, on the other hand, were not as knowledgeable about sexuality, and tended to describe activities such as cunnilingus in more graphic, objectifying detail. Men also acknowledged that they relied more heavily on pornography and firsthand experience when seeking information regarding female sexuality and felt substantially less comfortable seeking sex advice from parents and friends.

So where is a guy to go when seeking specific, accurate information regarding how to stimulate the process of female sexual response? The media bombards us with sex, 24/7, but there is very little mainstream discussion about human sexuality, and even less that is targeted specifically at men. Ironically, some of the guys I spoke with said that the television show *Sex and the City*—with its candid discussions of oral sex, orgasms, and other issues—was a principal source of information about women's sexual attitudes and desires. Still others confided that reading magazines like *Cosmo* and *Glamour* in private was illuminating, and that there was a quality of information that couldn't be found in men's magazines.

One guy summed it up: "*Cosmo* and *Glamour* are much more specific about sex and relationships than men's magazines like *Playboy* and *Maxim*, which constantly talk about sex, but not sexuality. They're more 'conquest-oriented' than advice-oriented, and they also focus a lot on gadgets, weight lifting, and getting ahead in your job. *Men's Health* definitely raises the bar, but that's just one magazine, and even it tends to focus more on achieving perfect abs than on detailed sex advice."

Unfortunately, both men *and* women end up suffering from this dearth of accurate information—with men flicking their tongues like porno stars, employing sexual positions that have little to do with clitoral stimulation, and generally being clueless about the female anatomy and the process of sexual response.

Why I Wrote this Book

My own education as a "cunnilinguist" began with sexual dysfunction—a long-drawn-out battle with premature ejaculation (PE). I was hopeless, pathetic. Just the sight of a woman's naked body could make me lose control, and foreplay quickly led to end of play. In the language of love, I couldn't get past the first syllable. I was sure that on my gravestone, my epitaph would read, "He came. He saw. And then he came again."

Later in life, I learned from my study of the pioneering sex researcher Alfred Kinsey that the typical male sustains penetrative thrusting, on average, for about two and a half minutes. That provided some small comfort, but at the time I felt terribly alone. I often wondered why I was "biologically cursed" to reach orgasm so quickly. Was it a vestigial remnant of the evolutionary battles of natural selection, when a man had to spread his seed quickly in order to ensure the propagation of his genetic material? Would Charles Darwin have told me that what I considered a grievous weakness was, in fact, a competitive advantage in the struggle for the survival of the fittest? Perhaps, but to me it felt more like the "barely hanging on of the unluckiest."

I was a sexual cripple, and oral sex became my crutch. If I couldn't satisfy a woman with my penis, then I'd sure as hell satisfy her with my mouth! I can still remember all the fears, preconceptions, and blunders of my early experiences in college. My first forays into cunnilingus were not unlike many men's—hesitant, tentative. I learned through trial and error, but eventually came to realize that cunnilingus was much more than just an arbitrary, or optional, aspect of foreplay; it was *coreplay*. It was an essential process—with a beginning, middle, and end—for leading a woman through the many stages of arousal that eventually culminate in orgasm. Cunnilingus not only enabled me to pleasure a woman utterly and completely, it allowed me to stop worrying about sex and start enjoying it. In doing so, I was able to drop the anxiety, develop greater self-control, and become a better lover overall. Cunnilingus certainly saved my sex life, and when I think about all the depression and heartache I suffered as a result of my battles with PE, it's not so far off to say that it saved my *entire* life.

I'll never forget the first time I ushered a woman into orgasm with my tongue. It was a watershed moment. I felt as E. B. White did when, recalling his years as a young struggling writer in New York, he described how it felt to sit down for dinner at Child's restaurant on Fourteenth Street and, going through his mail, discover his first check for a magazine piece he had written: "I can still remember the feeling that this was it, I was a pro at last. It was a good feeling and I enjoyed the meal."

I couldn't agree more.

Today, I'm happily married and able to make love successfully, but I still believe wholeheartedly in the "way of the tongue." It's simply the tool best suited for the job. More than that, I believe that cunnilingus is the most intimate, respectful, and rewarding sexual act a man can engage in. As Sally Tisdale wrote, "To submit to another's belly, or another's mouth. Oral sex may be the most potent of sexual acts. It is an act of power derived from the most vulnerable kind of intimacy."

Some people refer to oral sex as mouth-music, and as a musician I guess you can say I'm well down the path of accomplishment. But it wasn't until I met my wife that I found my Stradivarius—unique, beautiful, and priceless. If she is my violin, then I am her bow. I encourage you to find your Stradivarius. And when you do, protect, cherish, and remain constant to it, for then you will be able to play as a master.

As much as I will discuss general techniques for success, every woman is different, and cunnilingus is ultimately about individual acts of knowing and giving. That's not to say you can't have a lot of fun casually, but such exploits are ultimately the pursuit of technique without a greater sense of purpose—pyrotechnics rather than real fireworks. Giving great head requires trusting the rhythm of what happens and relaxing into a deeper, more instinctive zone of the self. It involves a mutual process of letting go and connecting to each other on every level. There's no faking it. You need to be more than just a technician. You need to imbue technique with all of your senses and imagination. You need to be present, you need to be real; you need to be there in body, mind, and spirit.

As E. B. White wrote, "Style results more from what a person is than from what he knows. But there are a few hints that can be thrown out to advantage."

With that in mind, let's get going.

PART

The Elements of Sexual Style

ONE

*"Following then the order of nature
let us begin with the principles which come first."*

—Aristotle, *Poetics*

She Comes First:
The Courtesy That Counts

L ADIES FIRST, gentlemen. When it comes to satisfying a woman, a little old-fashioned chivalry goes a long way.

Lest you think the importance of such courtesy is overexaggerated, direct your attention to Lorena Bobbitt, who when questioned by police as to why she cut off her husband's penis, responded, "He always has an orgasm and doesn't wait for me. It's unfair."

Need one say more?

Men are designed for efficiency. It doesn't often take much to get us aroused, and we tend to orgasm only once before requiring a "refractory period" (also known as the part where we turn over and start snoring). And depending upon our age, this period could last anywhere from a couple of minutes to a couple of days.

The simple fact is that in general male orgasms come easy. Masters and Johnson dubbed it "ejaculatory inevitability" and the late Dr. Alfred C. Kinsey, famous for interviewing thousands about their sex lives, declared that 75 percent of men ejaculate within two minutes.

But when it comes to the female orgasm, nothing's inevitable. As Sally Tisdale wrote:

> Male sexuality seems different from mine fundamentally because nothing need be involved but the head and shaft of the penis, no other part of the body need be troubled, touched, undressed, or soiled . . . the male orgasm has always seemed to me to burst almost from nowhere, to be infinitely more ready and willing than my own.

The female orgasm is a more complex affair and often takes much longer to achieve during a session of sexual activity. In particular, her first orgasm is the most difficult to accomplish, requiring persistent stimulation, concentration, and relaxation. Is it any surprise, then, that researchers from the University of Chicago declared in the 1994 *Sex in America Survey* that men reach orgasm during intercourse far more consistently than do women, and that three fourths of men, but less than a third of women, always have orgasms. Less than a third! That means more than two out of three women on average are consistently denied—good reason to start hiding the cutlery.

"The male belongs to Yang
Yang's peculiarity is that he is easily aroused.
But also he easily retreats.
The female belongs to Yin.
Yin's peculiarity is that she is slow to be aroused
But also slow to be satiated."
                    (Taoist master Wu Hsien)

Irony, bitter and cruel, seems to be embedded into our respective processes of arousal: that a woman, so unique in her sexuality, possessing both a clitoris—an organ designed solely for the production of pleasure—as well as the ability to experience multiple orgasms during a single session of sexual activity, should so often find this vast potential for blazing ecstasy smoldered—a magnificent conflagration left unlit—all for lack of a match that can hold its flame.

It's not a problem with the match, say many men, but rather that a woman's fuse is too long. Perhaps, but then this raises the question how long is too long? Studies, like those by Kinsey and Masters and Johnson, have concluded that among women whose partners spent twenty-one minutes or longer on foreplay, only 7.7 percent failed to reach orgasm consistently. That's a shift of tectonic proportions—from two out of three women *not* being able to reach climax to nine out of ten achieving satisfaction—all because of a matter of minutes.

Few, if any, of the world's problems can be solved with a mere twenty minutes of attention, and yet here, in the complex sociopolitical landscape of the bedroom, we have an opportunity to create bilateral satisfaction. When put that way, in the context of sexual peace and equality, is twenty minutes of focused attention, *applied appropriately*, really too much to ask, especially if it can save your sex life?

Take the path of the true gentleman: postpone your pleasure. As Sir Thomas Wyatt, father of the English sonnet wrote, "Patience shall be my song."

Ushering a woman into orgasm is both exhilarating and liberating. When she comes first, anxiety and pressure are dispensed with; you are emboldened, empowered to pursue with gusto the gratification that awaits you—a climax that will be heightened all the more for having been postponed.

I love to make my girlfriend come, I love to experience the whole thing—the buildup and release of waves of pleasure, the surrender to ecstasy, the spasm of satisfaction, the momentary loss of self. It turns me on even more to know I made it happen." (David, 27)

What greater reward could a man ask for?

Her Clitoris: The Little Engine
That Could

ILLUSION: The clitoris is "a tiny love button," "a little pink pearl," "small as a pea," "a bud," "a nub," "a nib," "a knob," "a teeny-weeny cock."

ALLUSION: There's more to the clitoris than meets the eye. Much more. Don't mistake the hooded crown (the "glans" or "head") for the entire clitoris. As we will discuss, the head is just the tip of the iceberg, a tantalizing allusion to unseen wells of pleasure. [1]

Like a Greek column, the clitoris has three components—a head,

[1]It's worth noting that within the medical and scientific communities the actual anatomy of the female clitoris is still a matter of some debate. While there exists a contingent of traditionalists who maintain that the clitoris is composed of nothing more than the glans (the head), there is also a more progressive and widely accepted view that builds on the research of pioneers like Masters and Johnson, Mary Jane Sherfey, and the Feminist Women's Health Centers among others. This view (espoused within these pages as well) maintains that the clitoris is a complex organ system that is homologous to the male penis.

a shaft, and a base—that extend throughout the pelvic area, with visible structures encompassing the entire area of the vulva, from the top of the pubic bone down to the anus, as well as unseen parts inside the vaginal area. In their landmark work, A New View of a Woman's Body: A Fully Illustrated Guide, the Federation of Feminist Women's Health Centers identified eighteen structures in the clitoral network, some visible, some hidden.

With more than eight thousand nerve fibers, the clitoris has more of these than any other part of the human body and interacts with the fifteen thousand nerve fibers that service the entire pelvic area. This vast erogenous landscape literally throbs with potential pleasure. As science writer Natalie Angier writes of the clitoral network, "Nerves are like wolves or birds: if one starts crying, there goes the neighborhood." So stop thinking of the clitoris as a little bump, and start thinking of it as a complex network, a pleasure dome, the Xanadu at the heart of female sexuality.

Because it's all that and more. When engorged with blood during sexual arousal, the clitoris increases in size, just like a penis. In fact, the clitoris was created from the same embryonic tissue as the penis, and can be compared point by point with the male genitalia. And unlike the penis—burdened with the responsibilities of reproduction and the removal of waste—the clitoris is devoted solely to pleasure and confers upon the female "an infinitely greater capacity for sexual response than a man ever dreamed of." (Masters and Johnson) According to Greek mythology, when Zeus and Hera went to the hermaphrodite Tiresias in order to determine who experiences more pleasure from sex, men or women, Tiresias responded, "If the sum of love's pleasure adds up to ten—nine parts go to women, only one to men."

Like Christopher Columbus sallying forth into the unknown, your exploration of the clitoral network will lead to the discovery of a whole new world. But knowing a little geography goes a long way. The earth isn't flat; nor is the clitoris a love button. Know your maps, and know that every voyage is unique.

Think Outside Her Box

WHEN DESCRIBING SEX in the proverbial locker room, men tend to employ the language of penetration—adjectives like "hard" and "deep." We go in, we extricate: "I screwed the _____ out of her"—as though pleasure was something buried deep inside her womb, a nugget to be rammed, jostled, and liberated with the powerful male tool.

Rare is the man who says, "I made love to her as subtly and lightly as a feather"; "I grazed her vulva as with the delicate wings of a butterfly"; "I barely touched her she came so hard!" And yet such language would be more appropriate, as the inner two thirds of the vagina are substantially less sensitive than the outer third. In a series of experiments, Dr. Kinsey asked five gynecologists to examine the genitals of almost nine hundred women in order to find out which areas were the most sensitive. "The deep interior walls of the vagina really have few nerve endings and are quite insensitive when stroked or lightly pressed." But when gently touched on their clitorises, 98 percent of women were aware of it.

The superiority of the clitoris to the vagina in stimulating the process of female sexual response is enough to throw many a guy into a tailspin and make him question the very meaning of life, or at least the meaning of his penis. But as difficult as it may be, it's important to separate the concept of procreation from pleasure: the penis, by dint of its convenient fit into the vagina, may play an instrumental role in the former, but that doesn't mean it's ideally suited to the latter.

This sort of talk is none too popular, mainly because it challenges the very foundation upon which our society's conception of sex has been forged, and throws into doubt the value of intercourse as the principal paradigm for constructing a model of mutual pleasure. From losing one's virginity to the consummation of a relationship to the cherished simultaneous orgasm, our culture has enshrined the role of genital penetration as the be-all, end-all of heterosexual relationships. Where would the "third date" be without it?

The idea that genital penetration might be seriously overhyped is a bitter pill to swallow, especially for those men of the world who base much of their sexual self-esteem on the value of their penis in stimulating female pleasure. As we will soon see, there is a long history of "clitoral denial" in our culture that stems back to Freud—a way of thinking so deeply embedded into our collective consciousness that even a woman is more likely to question, or repress, the natural instincts, responses, and sensations of her own body—or just fake her way through it—than to challenge the conventional wisdom or risk bruising the male ego. Is it any wonder, then, that according to author Lou Paget the number one question sent in by female readers to the editors of *Cosmopolitan* magazine is: What can I do to have an orgasm during intercourse? Here's a simple answer: Don't have intercourse. Or at least make it part of a larger event and not the event itself.

The pill doesn't have to be bitter, and once swallowed, it can be incredibly liberating. When we know how to recognize and navigate the process of female sexual response, when we understand the role of the clitoris in stimulating that process, then sex becomes easier, simpler, and more rewarding, and we're impelled to create pleasure not just with our penises, but with our hands and mouths, bodies and minds. In letting go of intercourse, we open ourselves up to new creative ways of experiencing pleasure, ways that may not strike us as inherently masculine, but ultimately allow us to be more of a man. Sex is no longer penis-dependent, and we can let go of the usual anxieties about size, stamina, and performance. We are free to love with more of ourselves, with our entire self.

The Female Orgasm: Keep it Simple

IN THE LORE of female sexuality, a lot of fuss is made over the differences between clitoral, G-spot, and blended and vaginal orgasms. The clitoral orgasm is often criticized as being quick and lighthearted, while the others are somehow deemed more serious and substantial. But a quick study of anatomy reveals that *all* orgasms are clitoral. The clitoris is the sexual epicenter, an orgasmic powerhouse in which no sensation goes unnoticed. As Natalie Angier writes of the infamous G-spot, the area of soft tissue just inside the vaginal area, "The roots of the clitoris run deep, after all, and very likely can be tickled through posterior agitation. In other words, the G-spot may be nothing more than the back end of the clitoris."

As for vaginal orgasms and the moans of pleasure that often accompany penetration, sorry to burst your bubble, gentlemen: while we'd like to believe that these sensations of excruciating ecstasy are being delivered from the depths of her vagina by the sheer power and reach of our formidable thrusts, they are actually "caused by pressure on the parts of the clitoris that surround the vaginal opening," what author Rebecca Chalker refers to as the "clitoral cuff." When this highly sensitized area is aroused and engorged with blood, a horseshoelike arch forms at the vaginal opening and applies friction and pressure against the male penis, playing a pivotal role in the stimulation of the male orgasm. So, in one sense, both the female *and* the male orgasm depend on the clitoris for stimulation.

For those doubting Thomases who still can't let go of their vaginal attachment, consider that an estimated one in five thousand women suffers from an unusual congenital disorder called vaginal agenesis, in which they are literally born *without* a vagina, despite normal development of external genitals, including major and minor labia. While these women are often unable to become pregnant without surgery or intense medical therapy, they are, in fact, *able to experience sexual pleasure and orgasm*—because even though they may lack a vagina, they still have a fully functional clitoris. Unfortunately, the same cannot be said of women who have been subjected to the brutalities of a clitoridectomy. This painful mutilation, often referred to as female circumcision, is still practiced today in some cultures and almost always leaves the woman permanently disfigured, traumatized, and deprived of a clitoris and any chance of sexual enjoyment.

What these two examples demonstrate is that even if one adamantly subscribes to the idea of vaginal and G-spot orgasms as being discrete orgasmic experiences unto themselves, the clitoris is clearly the "starter" or catalyst for sexual response. While it's possible to experience a clitoral orgasm without the presence of a vagina, it's virtually impossible to experience a vaginal or G-spot orgasm without the presence of a clitoris.

So when considering all of the various terms and types of female orgasm that are often bandied about, we can simplify matters by adopting "Occam's razor," the principle coined by the medieval philosopher William of Occam that lies at the root of all scientific modeling and theory building: *Entia non sunt multiplicanda necessitatem.* Translation: "One should not make more assumptions than are absolutely necessary."

When we speculate about the nature of a given phenomenon (like the female orgasm), this principle beseeches us to eliminate those concepts, variables, or constructs that are not needed to explain the phenomenon. In doing so, we reduce inconsistencies, ambiguities, and redundancies, as well as the likelihood of error.

So there's no need to quibble over semantics when it comes to identifying orgasms. The clitoris encompasses them all. The tongue is far better used to produce orgasms than to waste time naming them.

The Tongue Is Mightier
Than the Sword

NUMEROUS STUDIES have demonstrated that women whose lovers give them direct clitoral stimulation during sexual activity are more likely to climax consistently. But because of its location, most sexual positions (especially missionary-style) do not properly stimulate the clitoris. As Shere Hite concluded, "Sex provides efficiently for male orgasm, and inefficiently for female orgasm."

If you were going to paint a landscape in fine, subtle watercolors, would you use a soft, flexible brush, or a cumbersome, unwieldy roller? A woman's orgasm is complex and often elusive, and many men are unable to control their penises with enough precision to properly guide a woman through the stages of arousal. Making love with one's penis is like trying to write calligraphy with a thick Magic Marker.

The tongue, on the other hand, is under our direct control, has

I n *Sex: A Man's Guide* the authors conclude, "One of the biggest revelations of the *Men's Health* magazine survey was the num- ber of men who said that oral sex is the best way to ring her chimes. Over and over again, we heard such things as 'oral sex is the only method that consistently enables my wife to reach or- gasm' or 'if a man knows how to give outstanding oral sex, then a woman will reach orgasm every time.'"

no time constraints, and can be manipulated with expert precision. Unlike the penis, it's effective when hard or soft, and never gets overheated. When using his tongue, a man doesn't have to worry about growing fatigued, nor does he need fret over premature ejacu- lation or erectile disorder. He can relax and enjoy the act of giving.

The tongue, an array of muscles and nerves held together by a membrane covered with thousands of taste buds, is the most versa- tile sex organ we possess. It's the only muscle in the body that's not attached at both ends. We can touch, taste, and lick with it. The tongue is the instrument that lets us speak many languages, fore- most among them the language of love.

But having the right tool is just a start; you need to know how to use it. Many women complain woefully about men's oral tech- niques: the lack of consistent, rhythmic pressure; their roughness; the mad stampede for the clitoris. As Strunk and White wrote in *El- ements of Style*, "Do not overstate . . . a single overstatement, wher- ever or however it occurs, diminishes the whole."

Sadly, many women also complain about men's attitudes toward cunnilingus: squeamish and hesitant; overeager, impatient, even an- gry. And many men fail to finish what they started. In *The Hite Re- port on Male Sexuality*, the author observes that although most men enjoy cunnilingus, only a small minority of men continued to per- form it until the woman reached orgasm.

Most men consider cunnilingus an aspect of foreplay, an appetizer to be served before the main meal of genital intercourse. But according to author Paula Kamen, "In a study of sexually knowledgeable and experienced women who use a vibrator, the most common type of stimulation that usually or always triggers an orgasm is oral sex."

So perhaps we need to find a word other than "foreplay" in order to properly classify and appreciate the importance of cunnilingus. We need a category that is more encompassing and inclusive. Kamen cites a 1996 *Mademoiselle* article in which author Valerie Frankel uses the term "outercourse" to describe those important nongenital activities that frequently fall under the rubric of foreplay: "Women of the 90s are not squeamish little virgins. We've had intercourse—lots of it—and think that Outercourse kicks its ass."

Regardless of how we categorize it, we need to understand that cunnilingus is a complete process that takes a woman through the gamut of sexual response. Later, in Part II, cunnilingus will be referred to as *coreplay*—the centerpiece of the "play process"—with foreplay encompassing those activities prior to the first "genital kiss."

G iving expert cunnilingus requires learning appropriate techniques (through reading a book such as this and also through individual experimentation) and then applying them consistently over time in a focused, patient, and loving manner; most important, it requires respecting, sharing, and participating wholly in the erotic intimacy of the moment.

"The penis is very badly placed, anatomically speaking, when it comes to making women come. Better if men simply left their penis alone, stopped attending to those immature nerve fibers, and concentrated instead on learning how to orgasm through their tongues." (Tisdale)

It sounds funny, but in a certain sense we *can* orgasm through our tongues. It's not that the tongue is a replacement for the penis; if anything, it's an addition, an enhancement—an extension. Men often joke of having two heads, the big and the little, and of their frequent battles with each other. However, during cunnilingus, if you trust the moment and let yourself go, you enter a zone where *both* your heads are united in a process of arousal that is synchronized with hers. You become one with yourself and her.

Her Inner Goddess

IMAGINE A WORLD in which a woman's orgasm, along with the male's, is a necessary and *critical* part of the reproductive process: a world in which human beings can't reproduce unless *both* man and woman experience orgasm at the moment of insemination. In this bizarre world, men are selected as mates based not on their proficiency to wield a spear or look good in a tux, but on their ability to consistently lead a woman to climax; only those men who are able to experience their pleasure as part of a woman's find themselves accepted by society. The rest are ostracized, cast out, banished to the margin.

Sounds strange, like the makings of a Margaret Atwood novel or an X-rated episode of *The Twilight Zone*, but in fact, up through the eighteenth century, scientists, doctors, and philosophers believed that the female orgasm was an integral component of reproduction. As Natalie Angier noted, "The ancients also saw no difference between men's and women's capacity for sexual pleasure and the necessity of the female orgasm for conception. Galen proclaimed that a woman could not get pregnant unless she had an orgasm."

This type of "nonscientific" thinking hearkens back thousands of years, to a time before patriarchs, to an age of matriarchs and goddess worship, when societies revered a woman's sexuality as a life-giving force, and celebrated it with elaborate sex rituals that took place in temples and included costumes, incense, poetry, music, feasts, and wine.

We tend to take it for granted that our society defines sex as a linear process that includes foreplay, vaginal penetration, and the male orgasm. And because of its role in the act of procreation, the male orgasm/ejaculation is enshrined in our culture's definition of sex. The male orgasm presages the denouement of the sex act, regardless of where a woman is in the process of sexual response and irrespective of her innate biological capacity to experience multiple orgasms. The male orgasm is the signifying event that defines what comes before, as well as after. The male orgasm is indispensable and highly valued by society, not so the females.

What happened? Even up through the seventeenth century, Western science and society maintained a "one-sex" view of the human anatomy; that the genitals of men and women were similar and functioned in a similar way to produce orgasm. As long as the one-sex view prevailed, the capacity for female pleasure was understood, if not always respected.

According to Rebecca Chalker, author of the insightful book *The Clitoral Truth*, as Western civilization (and women's discontents) progressed through the eighteenth and nineteenth centuries, "Women's sexuality was seen as very different from men's—increasingly weak and chaste and passionless."

Chalker continues, "Anatomists began to ascribe parts of the clitoris to the reproductive or urinary system. Medical illustrations became increasingly more simplistic, leaving parts of the clitoris

unlabelled. By Victorian times, the orgasm, which was previously accepted as a natural component of women's sexual repertoire, was seen
as unnecessary, unseemly, and perhaps even unhealthy for women."

In the very first paragraph of his essay, "The Functions and Dis-
orders of the Reproductive Organs," the well-known Victorian
doctor William Acton stated, "I should say that the majority of
women (happily for society) are not very much troubled with sexual feelings of any kind. What men are habitually, women are only
exceptionally."

And then, as if the clitoris didn't have enough problems, along
came a psychoanalyst with a Big Cigar (and sometimes, regardless of
size, a cigar is really just a cigar) . . .

Avoid Freud

SIGMUND FREUD made a name for himself demonizing the clitoris and formulating a truly cockamamie view of women's sexuality. Freud promulgated the idea that the clitoris was an immature source of sexual pleasure, a mere launching pad for the more "mature" vaginal orgasm, which, of course, could only be produced via genital intercourse. What's particularly insidious is that at the time of his postulating Freud had a rather clear understanding of the anatomical role of the clitoris and chose instead to promote his personal ideas about female sexuality over current scientific knowledge.

Freud demoted the clitoris and promoted the vagina, characterizing clitoral orgasms as "infantile." According to Freud, adult women needed to get past their need for clitoral orgasms and develop a desire for penetration; after all, isn't that what penises do? Penetrate? Female masturbation was criticized as creating clitoral

W ith the change to femininity the clitoris should wholly, or in part, hand over its sensitivity and at the same time its importance to the vagina.

(Freud, *New Introductory Lectures on Psychoanalysis*)

dependency; cunnilingus was verboten. In Freud's view, there were no two ways about it: if a woman couldn't be satisfied by penetrative sex, something must be wrong with her. As Dr. Thomas Lowry commented in his essay "The Cultural Psychology of the Clitoris," "The idea sprang into Freud's head in 1910 without a visible shred of experimental evidence and it has probably caused more unnecessary worry than any other single psychological notion."

Since it was well known at the time that sensitive nerve endings contributing to sexual response were on the surface of a woman's genital area, Freud's views were not based on physiology, or an understanding of anatomy, but rather on a conception of human sexuality that reinforced the penetrative, reproductive model. Hence, a woman's sexuality became subsumed by a male's. From there, it was all downhill.

"Freud's summary dismissal of the clitoris as an important focus of sexual sensation for women had an atomic effect on how physicians and psychologists perceived women's sexuality. It was as if, for most of the twentieth century, women's extensive genital anatomy, and even the explosive little glans, was vaporized. Memory of the clitoris gradually faded until it became an anatomical nonentity." (Chalker)

Alas, if only Freud, who himself said "anatomy is destiny," had had the "clitoral sense" to see that this powerful organ would eventually rise from the ashes of his much-ballyhooed cigar. In fairness to Freud, it should be acknowledged that as he neared the end of his life he acknowledged his incomplete understanding of female sexuality and said, "If you want to know more about femininity, you must interrogate your own experience, or turn to the poets, or else wait until science can give you more profound and more coherent information."

Today, our understanding and appreciation of the importance of the clitoris, and the stimulation of it, owes much to the dogged efforts of those impassioned individuals who bucked the conventional wisdom and did battle throughout the sexual revolution of the 1950s, 1960s, and 1970s: prominent figures such as Dr. Alfred Kinsey, Masters and Johnson, Shere Hite, Betty Dodson, and less prominent, but equally important ones like Dr. Mary Jane Sherfey, who pioneered the idea that the clitoris is a powerful organ system.

But knowledge is only powerful when disseminated and put into practice. Men need to take the time to learn what most women know intuitively about their bodies—how to listen to and feel them—and sex needs to be redefined as an activity that accommodates a wide variety of sensual and erotic activities; including, but by no means limited to, genital intercourse.

In both philosophy and practice, any definition of sex must, first and foremost, include a powerful element of respect. According to journalist Paula Kamen, author of the survey of sexual attitudes *Her Way*, "Women receiving oral sex is an act most directly reflecting women's growing power in both their sexual relationships and in society. The practice depends on both women's and men's recognition and respect of this power."

In *The Cradle of Erotica* by A. Edwardes and R.E.L. Masters, we are told that during the Tang Dynasty, the Empress Wu Hu ruled China. She knew that sex and power were inexorably linked, and she

When my husband gives me head, it's such a powerful turn-on . . . he's completely focused on me, I'm the center of his attention, and I feel like he's really loving me, every part of me, all at once." (Kelly, 32)

decreed that government officials and visiting dignitaries must pay homage to her imperial highness by performing cunnilingus upon her. No joke. Old paintings depict the beautiful, powerful empress standing and holding her ornate robe open while a high nobleman or diplomat is shown kneeling before her, applying his lips and tongue to her royal mound.

Well gone are the days of kings and queens and royal decrees, but inside many a modern woman is an Empress Wu Hu, longing to be honored by her nobleman.

What's in a Name?

L ET'S FACE IT. Most men can more easily identify what's under the hood of a car than what's under the hood of a clitoris.
This "genital confusion" arises because parts of the clitoral network
are hidden from the naked eye. Even though the genitals of both
men and women are formed from the same embryonic material, and
develop during gestation in an equivalent manner, the penis grows
out, while much of the clitoris grows *in*. (Interestingly, Oliver Wen-
dell Holmes remarked that the female genitalia were simply those of
the male turned inside out. But on the contrary, modern science
teaches us that the male is a modified female, differentiated during
the first trimester of pregnancy. So if anything, the male genitalia
are a mirror image of the female's rather than vice versa.)

"Vagina or Vulva: That Is the Question"

The visible parts of the female genitalia are encompassed by the vulva, or what's commonly, and mistakenly, referred to as the vagina. "Vagina" tends to be the de facto word we use to describe "everything down there," but the entrance to the vagina, also known as the "introitus," is just one part of the vulva's impressive expanse and certainly not the primary part when it comes to stimulation and the process of arousal.

Etymologically, "vagina" originates from a Latin word meaning "a sheath or scabbard for a sword," reinforcing its relationship to the penis and dependency upon penetration or insertion for broader meaning—which may be indicative of the reproductive process, but certainly not the pleasure process.

What's in a name? According to Shakespeare, "That which we call a rose by any other name would smell as sweet." But the language of science is by no means the language of love; "cunnilingus," "vulva," and "vaginal introitus"—those may not be the first words that come to mind in the heat of the moment. But they're the *right* words, in that they're scientifically accurate and properly descriptive. And knowing the right words is a powerful starting point for clearly understanding the process of sexual response and, ultimately, developing an erotic lexicon that is unique and true to the spirit of your individual relationship.

In speaking of *The Vagina Monologues*, author and activist Eve Ensler described her thought process in committing to the word "vagina" in both the title and throughout the work

> I say it because we haven't come up with a word that is more inclusive, that really describes the entire area and all its parts. . . . "Vulva" is a good word; it speaks more specifically, but I don't think most of us are clear what the vulva includes.

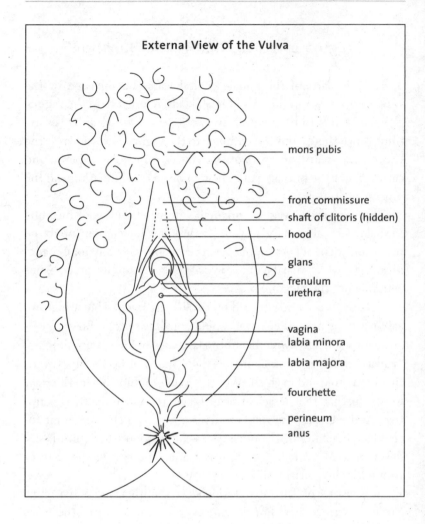

External View of the Vulva

mons pubis

front commissure

shaft of clitoris (hidden)

hood

glans

frenulum

urethra

vagina

labia minora

labia majora

fourchette

perineum

anus

Ms. Ensler is right: the term "vulva" is much more specific and inclusive, especially when describing the visible parts of the clitoris. Although the vagina plays an extremely active role in the reproductive process, it takes a backseat to the clitoris in the production of pleasure; employing "vagina" as a catchall phrase for describing a woman's genitalia actually promotes an inaccurate understanding of female anatomy, perhaps even more so than the more generic "down there."

So, "vulva" it is—in the interest of accuracy, as well as in the hope of promoting greater familiarity with the term. The words you choose to use in your bedroom are your own business; supplying you with accurate knowledge is this book's business.

Now You See It:
Female Sexual Anatomy Part 1

The Vulva and External Parts
of the Clitoris[2]

STARTING WITH the visible parts of the clitoral network, let's take a closer look at what's really "down there."

The Mons Pubis. We begin our journey, north, at the mons pubis, also known as the "mons veneris" (mountain of Venus), named after the Roman goddess of love. The mons pubis is a thick pad of fatty

---

[2]While there is no shortage of documentation on the female sexual anatomy, as well as on the process of female sexual response, our review of these areas is based on the groundbreaking work of the Federation of Feminist Women's Health Centers and their highly informative book A *New View of a Woman's Body*. Based on years of research and self-examination, FFWHC has redefined much of what had been previously held to be true about the nature of female sexuality.

Interestingly, the principal function of pubic hair is to attract and retain odors that stem from the release of glands in the pubic area and serve as a source of arousal. As Napoleon noted in a love letter to Josephine: "A thousand kisses to your neck, your breasts, and lower down, much lower down, that little black forest I love so well."

tissue, covered in pubic hair, which is sometimes called the love mound because it forms a soft mound over the pubic bone.

The Labia Majora. Heading south from the mons pubis, we next encounter the starting point of the labia majora (major lips). The outer sides of the labia majora, also known as the outer lips, are rich with pubic hair, whereas their inner sides are smooth, lined with oil and sweat glands. Beneath the skin of the outer lips is a network of erectile tissue that engorges with blood during arousal. The outer lips are analogous to the male scrotum, and both were formed from the same embryonic tissue. Although sensitive to touch, the outer lips are not nearly as sensitive as the labia minora (small lips) or other parts of the clitoral network such as the head and shaft.

The Front Commissure. The outer lips mark an area where the visible parts of the clitoris begin. This highly sensitive area, just above the clitoral head, is called the front commissure, and it's from this point that the clitoral shaft—an unseen, but instrumental part of the clitoris—protrudes.

The Labia Minora. Enfolded within the labia majora are the labia minora (little lips), although many insist that it's more apt to refer to both sets of lips respectively as *outer* and *inner*, rather than big and little, since the inner lips sometimes protrude out and beyond the outer lips. Interestingly, the inner lips are also archaically known

Some anthropologists speculate that a woman's use of lipstick stems from her desire to have the visible upper lips resemble the inner hidden lips below—a signal to the opposite sex that she is sexually ready.

as "nymphae," named after the nymphs of ancient Greece who were famous for their irrepressible libidos and are the source of the term "nymphomania."

The inner lips enfold and surround the clitoral glans (the head), the urethral opening, and the introitus (entrance) to the vagina. Like the inner side of the labia majora, these smaller, inner lips have no hair, but are layered with oil glands that look and feel like tiny bumps. Dense with nerves, the inner lips are extremely sensitive and play an important role in the process of arousal.

The inner lips are remarkably diverse in size and appearance. From woman to woman, and often on the *same* woman, no two lips are the same. Some lips are narrow; others wide; some curl inward, others flare outward. Sometimes the texture is glossy and smooth, sometimes wrinkled and bumpy. During the process of arousal, the inner lips change color, from light pink to darker hues, and swell and puff in size as they engorge with blood.

The Hood. The outer edges of the inner lips meet just above the sensitive clitoral head to form the well-known protective hood (which is analogous to the foreskin of the penis), also known as the prepuce. The friction created when the clitoral hood rubs against the head is a powerful source of stimulation and pleasure. The hood also protects the head from overstimulation; just prior to the release of orgasm, it's into the folds of the hood that the head seeks refuge.

The Frenulum. Below the head, the inner edges of the labia minora meet to form the frenulum, a small expanse of soft, sensitive skin, also known as the bridle. Like the inner lips, this area is rich in nerve fibers and is extremely sensitive to the touch.

The Fourchette. The bottom edges of the lips meet beneath the vaginal entrance in an area known as the fourchette, or little fork. Just as the front commisure marks the top part of the visible clitoris, the fourchette marks the bottom.

The Clitoral Glans (the head). Protected by the hood of the inner lips, the head is the crown jewel that rests atop the unseen shaft and crura (the legs). With approximately eight thousand nerve endings, twice as many as the head of the penis and more than any other part of the human body, the head is the visible part of a woman's clitoris that often gets referred to as the "love button." It's not a bad term; just remember that it applies to only *one* part of the clitoris—the head.

One of the biggest mistakes a lover can make is to underestimate the sensitivity of the clitoral head. In fact, at the peak of sexual arousal, the head becomes so sensitive that, with a little help from the suspensory ligament (an unseen part of the of the clitoris), it retracts beneath its hood and is often hidden at the moment of climax.

Some heads are large; others are small. Size varies greatly, just as it does with the male penis. But regardless of size and shape, all contain the same number of nerve endings, so clitoral dimensions have no impact on a woman's sensitivity.

There's quite a bit of contention over the etymology of the word "clitoris." Some believe it stems from the Greek, *kleitoris*, meaning "little hill or slope"; others say it comes from the Greek verb *kleitoriazein*, meaning "to touch or titillate lasciviously, to be inclined to pleasure"; and still others claim that the Greek word *kleitoris* originally meant "divine and goddesslike." In some sense, all these meanings are true.

Perineum. The perineum is the small expanse of skin just above the anus and just beneath the vaginal entrance (sometimes referred to

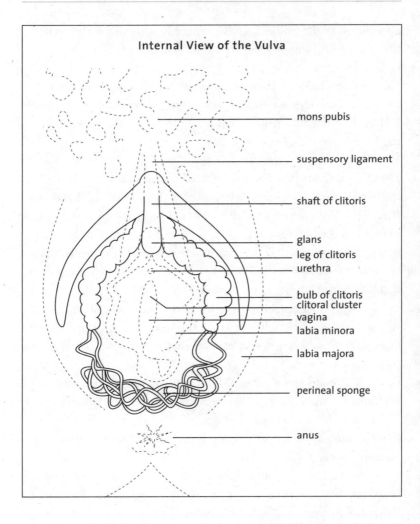

Internal View of the Vulva

mons pubis

suspensory ligament

shaft of clitoris

glans
leg of clitoris
urethra

bulb of clitoris
clitoral cluster
vagina
labia minora

labia majora

perineal sponge

anus

casually as the "taint," because "it t'aint one or the other"). Beneath the skin of the perineum is a network of blood vessels and tissue, which fill with blood during arousal and become intensely sensitive. Dr. Kinsey observed during his research that the perineum is "highly sensitive to touch, and tactile stimulation of the area may provide considerable erotic arousal." When making your travel plans of the clitoral network, make sure to include this southern hot spot.

10
Now You Don't:
Female Sexual Anatomy Part 2

The Internal Parts of
the Clitoris

WHEN IT COMES to the female genitalia and the hidden parts of the clitoris, seeing is only the first part of believing. You need to rely on all of your senses, especially touch. In their book *A New View of a Woman's Body*, the Feminist Center for Health identified eighteen parts in the clitoral network, many of which are unseen but are nonetheless felt or contribute to the experience of feeling. Let's review the internal parts of the clitoris:

The Clitoral Body. Attached to the head, and running just beneath the surface of the skin, the clitoral shaft can easily be felt, especially when aroused and filled with blood. A soft little pipe, the shaft is composed of spongy erectile tissue that is extremely receptive to sensation. The shaft extends north from the head toward the mons pubis for about three quarters of an inch before forking and dividing like a wishbone into two thin crura (or legs) that flare downward along the path of the inner lips and surround twin bulbs of erectile tissue, known as the clitoral bulbs.

If you've ever noticed that the clitoral head seems to retract and disappear under its protective hood during peak arousal, that's because the suspensory ligament—attached to the head at one end and the ovaries at the other—is being stretched, causing the head to retract.

Additionally, the clitoris has layers of muscle, usually referred to as vaginal muscles or pelvic floor muscles. There is the oval-shaped bulbocavernous muscle that rests between the inner lips and the bulbs of the clitoris. This muscle is interwoven with muscle that encircles the anus, and is part of the reason that anal stimulation is often a turn-on and hence part of the clitoral network.

Underneath it all is a broad, flat layer of muscle called the pubococcygeus (pew-bo-cok-SIH-gee-us) or PC muscle. The PC muscle is also known as the "Kegel" muscle, named after Dr. Arnold Kegel who observed that the PC muscle contracts during orgasm. Kegel subsequently developed a series of exercises designed to strengthen the pelvic muscles and heighten pleasure for both partners, hence the birth of "Kegels." In both men and women, the PC muscle is easily identified as the one that allows us to stop the flow of urine.

Avoid "G-Spotty" Logic

L ET'S TALK about spot removal, G-spot removal that is. Starting at the urethral opening, and running about two inches deep to the bladder, is the urethra, which first and foremost enables the removal of urine. Surrounding the urethra is a ring of spongy erectile tissue, known as corpus spongiosum, which fills with blood during arousal and protects the urethra from the friction of penetration. This area of spongy tissue is also known as the G-spot, named in 1944 after Dr. Ernst Grafenberg, who described a "zone of erogenous feeling . . . located along the suburethral surface of the anterior vaginal wall." In layman's terms, Dr. Kinsey observed, "Most of those women who did notice some response had the sensitivity confined to a certain point, in most cases the upper wall of the vagina just inside the vaginal entrance." For all its hype, the G-spot, as cited earlier, may simply be nothing more than the roots of the clitoris crisscrossing the urethral sponge.

While sensitive to stimulation, but without nearly as many nerve endings as the clitoral head, the G-spot generally responds to a more persistent, massaging pressure. It's not uncommon for a woman to feel a fleeting urge to urinate when this area is stimulated.

A whole lot of fuss has been made over the difference between a clitoral orgasm and a G-spot orgasm, with many claiming that the latter is responsible for the production of the fuller vaginal orgasm. This hubbub reached its apex with the publication in 1982 of the *The G Spot* by Alice Kahn Ladas, Beverly Whipple, and Dr. John Perry. In retrospect, it's possible to argue that their book ultimately reintroduced a spruced-up, hyped-up theory of vaginal orgasm into the mainstream, with the added bonus of female ejaculation. Of course it was a cultural sensation; the notion of a G-spot dovetailed seamlessly into the "intercourse discourse" and gave penetration a new, invigorated raison d'être.

As we discussed earlier, the whole idea of a *mature* vaginal orgasm vs. an *immature* clitoral one was a bogus construct to begin with, promulgated by Freud, perpetuated by his followers, and reinvented and sensationalized in the form of the G-spot. And although the urethral sponge is indeed attached to the vaginal ceiling, it is nevertheless considered an integral part of the clitoral network and not a separate part of the vagina that produces pleasure. A G-spot orgasm, like all female orgasms, is a clitoral orgasm; it's part of the same pleasure network. As such, when we address the techniques in Part II, this book will make a somewhat radical break from the tradition of erotological literature by referring to the area that is generally known as the G-spot as the "clitoral cluster," a name that more accurately, and simply, expresses its anatomical power and role in the process of female sexual response.

When Raindrops Keep Falling
on Your Head: Female Ejaculation

THE G-SPOT, or clitoral cluster, is also thought to be the source of female ejaculation, another matter of controversy. Does a woman actually ejaculate? The answer is yes, but not in the same sense as the explosive male orgasm and not nearly as often as the "ejaculation evangelists" would have us believe. In general, female ejaculation appears to be the exception rather than the rule. Today, a whole industry has emerged around the concept, pitching a vast array of books, tapes, videos, and seminars that urge women to discover and master their ejaculatory potential. But it's worth keeping in mind that the orgasm reflex is part of the autonomic nervous system—it's an involuntary response outside of the control of the mind. The momentary out-of-body sense of "timelessness" that we experience when we've reached the point of no return is intrinsic to the release of sexual tension and part and parcel of the joy of sexual ecstasy; it shouldn't be muddled up with mind-control exercises

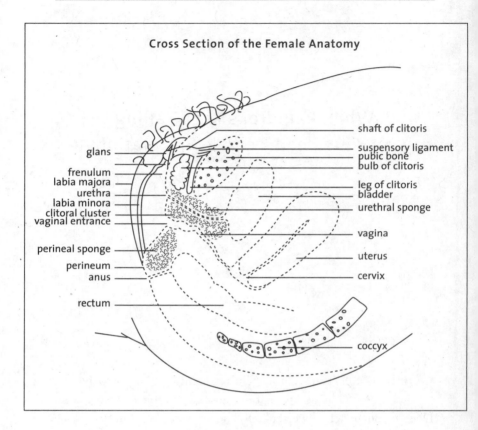

Cross Section of the Female Anatomy

glans

frenulum
labia majora
urethra
labia minora
clitoral cluster
vaginal entrance

perineal sponge

perineum
anus

rectum

shaft of clitoris

suspensory ligament
pubic bone
bulb of clitoris

leg of clitoris
bladder

urethral sponge

vagina

uterus

cervix

coccyx

that may, in the end, enable a woman to produce a bit of fluid, but do not qualitatively enhance the experience of orgasm, and indeed may ultimately detract from it.

Where does female ejaculate come from? Depends on what type of emission you're talking about. The type of fluid that sometimes gets released as part of the natural involuntary orgasmic reflex appears to originate in the area of spongy tissue that surrounds the urethra and encompasses tiny para-urethral glands. Two of the largest of these glands are called Skene's glands and appear near the urethral opening. Some studies have argued that the fluid produced by these glands is actually urine. Upon analysis, however, it's been concluded that these glands, in fact, produce a clear alkaline fluid that is much closer in composition to male prostatic fluid, and gives rise to the even more controversial notion of the existence of a female prostate. In fact, until 1880, these para-urethral glands were simply called "prostates." In short, female ejaculate of this sort is *not* urine.

However, the fluid that is reputed to gush when consciously impelled by the bearing down of the pelvic muscles may very well be coming from the bladder and thereby contain urine. Women who train themselves to consciously ejaculate also appear to produce more fluid than women who emit fluid involuntarily, lending further credence to the idea that urine may be contributing to the overall volume of ejaculate. What's interesting as well is that interviews with women who are able to voluntarily ejaculate reveal that the process is independent of sexual arousal and does not necessarily heighten the pleasure of orgasm, whereas women who involuntarily ejaculate are unable to parse the experience of orgasm and ejaculation and often don't even know that they've ejaculated.

All in all, it does not appear that female ejaculation, voluntary or involuntary, does much to enhance the pleasure of orgasm. To that end, a woman's time would be better spent on Kegel exercises and the strengthening of the pelvic floor muscles—an exercise known to increase the quality of orgasmic contractions.

How Wet Is Wet?

IN A NONAROUSED STATE, the vagina is a compressed tube, about three to four inches long, composed of muscle, and lined with mucous membranes not dissimilar to the lining of the mouth. During arousal, a woman's vagina widens and opens in order to accommodate the penis—a few inches in both depth and width—creating what Masters and Johnson referred to as the "ballooning" effect. Meanwhile, the outer third of the vagina begins to narrow and tighten as the clitoral structures that are located there fill with blood; this compression creates a "clitoral cuff" that actually helps stimulate a man to orgasm through the application of pressure and friction against the penis.

A woman's vagina usually begins to lubricate shortly after stimulation—what looks like beads of sweat form all over the vaginal walls; this is sometimes called vaginal sweating. Just below the vaginal opening are the ducts that connect to the vulvovaginal glands,

In Taoist sex practices, a woman's vaginal secretions are considered an essential part of her "yin" energy, a libation that should be savored in the pursuit of yin/yang harmony and is referred to as "moon flower."

which secrete a few drops of thick fluid that contribute, along with the sweating of the vagina, to the lubrication of the vaginal opening.

As we will discuss in the section on foreplay, lubrication is a big part of the arousal process, but is by no means an unequivocal indicator that a woman's been amply stimulated. She may be lubricated, but not necessarily aroused. These secretions are part of the vagina's natural way of keeping it free of bacteria that don't belong there. Conversely, a woman may be highly aroused, yet not necessarily well lubricated.

In short, a woman's ability to lubricate can be impacted by a variety of factors—her estrogen levels, diet, and stress to name a few. And while lubrication is connected to the process of arousal and plays an important role in subsequent sexual activity, assessing her readiness for sex depends on a variety of factors and is ultimately more art than science.

Now that we've met the various parts of the clitoral network—both visible and hidden—let's take a closer look at how they interact and come together in the process of sexual response. Again we take our cue from Strunk and White: "Before beginning to compose something, gauge the nature and extent of the enterprise, and work from a suitable design . . . you cannot plunge in blindly . . . lest you miss the forest for the trees and there be no end to your labors."

Summary of the 18 Parts of the Clitoris

In *The Clitoral Truth*, author Rebecca Chalker delineates the eighteen parts of the clitoris based on the research of the Federation of Feminist Women's Health Centers. Here's an abridged version. (Don't let the list overwhelm you; in Part II, we'll take a much closer look at the important hot-spots, one by one, and soon they'll be right on the tip of your tongue.)

1. The front commissure (the point where the outer lips meet at the base of the mons pubis).
2. The glans (head).
3. The inner lips, or labia minora.
4. The clitoral hood.
5. The frenulum (the point where the outer edges of the inner lips meet just below the head).
6. The fourchette (the point where the inner lips meet beneath the vaginal opening).
7. The hymen, or its remnants, visible just inside the vaginal opening.
8. The clitoral shaft, which connects the head and the legs.
9. The legs, or crura, two elongated bodies of erectile tissue, shaped like a wishbone.
10. The bulbs, two large bodies of spongy erectile tissue.
11. The urethral sponge, or G-spot (attached to the vaginal ceiling).
12. The para-urethral glands: the female prostate glands that produce ejaculate.
13. The vulvovaginal glands, which produce a small amount of lubricant outside of the vagina.
14. The perineal sponge, a dense network of blood vessels that lies underneath the perineum.

15. The pelvic floor muscles.
16. The suspensory ligament and round ligament.
17. The pudendal nerve, or genital nerve complex,* which carries messages up the spinal cord, between the brain and clitoris.
18. The blood vessels, which increase blood supply to the pelvic area during arousal and engorge the erectile tissues, causing them to swell.

*The original meaning of the Latin word *pudendum* is "a source of shame," and so Chalker redubbed this part of the clitoral network in more positive, accurate terms. Many, including this author, believe that "pudenda" is an antiquated word that should be left to antiquity.

Aristotle and the Poetics
of Arousal

"OUR PRINCIPLES being established let us now discuss the proper structure of the Plot, since this is the first and most important thing."

Twenty-five hundred years ago, the Greek philosopher Aristotle delineated in his timeless work *Poetics* the fundamental elements of Greek tragedy and much of what we understand today to be the essence of narrative storytelling.

Like a great work of dramatic literature, there's a structure to the process of arousal; a narrative that encompasses a beginning, middle, and end, with each element taking its natural place in the overall sequence of events. The parts of the clitoral network that we met in the preceding chapters are like actors in a drama that interact and make their entrances and exits according to the cues of the larger script.

Aristotle emphasized the importance of plot: the call to action that sets into motion a series of events that unfold over time in a unified, organic manner; the driving force that defies chaos and governs the arrangement of scenes; the structure that confers order and reason upon the various parts and weaves them together into an organized whole—"that which has a beginning, middle, and an end. Most important of all is the structure of the incidents. If any one of them is displaced or removed, the whole will be disjointed and disturbed."

In the drama of arousal, body and mind are called to action, sexual tension develops and builds to a peak, climax occurs, and then relaxation ensues. Masters and Johnson called this sequence the "sexual response cycle," while sex researchers Beverly Whipple and Barry Komisaruk called it the "orgasmic process"; each described the unfolding of an almost procedural series of events, with each successive step dependent on the satisfactory completion of the one that comes before it. Masters and Johnson broke down the process of sexual response into four stages: Excitement, Plateau, Orgasm, and Resolution. With the application of steady, rhythmic stimulation, each phase builds upon the last in the creation and release of sexual tension.

In Part II, the section of this book dedicated to specific techniques, we will refer to the journey through sexual response as the "play process," one that encompasses three distinct stages: foreplay, coreplay, and moreplay.

With that in mind, let's move on to a synopsis of sexual response.

A Synopsis of Female
Sexual Response

Act I—Foreplay: The Call to Action

I N ACT I, foreplay galvanizes the mind and body toward sexual response.

- Dozens of chemicals and hormones are released into the bloodstream, causing a woman to become "emotionally stoned," according to Theresa Crenshaw, M.D., author of *The Alchemy of Love and Lust.*
- The flow of blood is redirected toward the pelvic area; nerve fibers in the genital area become excited, and erectile tissue begins to engorge.
- Across the body, the skin becomes extra sensitive to touch.
- The breasts swell in size, and stimulation of the nipples ini-

tiates the production of oxytocin, a hormone that creates pleasurable sensations throughout the genital area.

- As blood vessels force fluid through the walls of the vagina, the vulvovaginal glands produce a small amount of thick fluid that acts as a lubricant.
- The clitoral head emerges from its hood.

Act II—Coreplay: Tension and Release

- Muscle tension builds throughout the body, respiration increases, blood pressure goes up, and the heart beats faster.
- The entrance to the vagina narrows while its inner depths widen and increase at least two inches in length.
- The clitoral body (the shaft, legs, and bulb) stiffens, stretches, and elongates.
- The spongy tissue of the clitoral cluster swells and its ridges can be clearly felt protruding from the vaginal ceiling.
- The suspensory ligament tightens and causes the highly sensitized clitoral head to retract beneath its hood, where it will remain until orgasm.
- The round ligament, positioned between the uterus and the inner lips, tugs on both ends, involving the uterus in the process of sexual response and climax.

As coreplay continues:

- The skin flushes; breathing deepens.
- The heart rate soars, everything tightens in a final clench.

During the process of arousal, erectile tissue engorges with blood, causing the clitoral head nearly to double in size.

- Her inner labia change color, darkening with the engorgement of blood.

Finally, all the muscular tension that has been building explodes in orgasm—a series of quick, rhythmic contractions.

- The vagina walls and the pelvic floor muscles contract rhythmically in approximately 0.8-second intervals.
- The sphincter muscles in the rectum also contract spasmodically in sync with genital contractions. In addition, the uterus contracts from an influx of oxytocin.
- These contractions produce waves of pleasure, and with some women the orgasm is accompanied by the ejaculation of a small amount of clear, alkaline fluid.

The number of orgasmic contractions varies, anywhere from three to fifteen on average, although Masters and Johnson observed a woman who experienced a forty-three-second orgasm consisting of more than twenty-five successive contractions. Additionally, it's been observed that pregnant women sometimes experience prolonged orgasms because of the persistent engorgement of their genitals.

While the orgasm originates from the genital area, it is often experienced and felt throughout the body. Every woman's orgasm is

While there's no rule of thumb for the number of orgasmic contractions, women tend to experience six to ten contractions, whereas men generally have four to six. Once again, we are reminded of Masters and Johnson's declaration that a woman has "an infinitely greater capacity for sexual response than a man ever dreamed of."

different and highly individualized. Sex researchers often refer to this sense of uniqueness as "orgasmic fingerprinting."

There's a wonderful passage in Norman Rush's novel *Mortals* in which the central character recounts his wife's description of an orgasm, or rather, in her words, "what it feels like when you come really hard":

> Well, part of what it feels like is this, that you're just a drop of oil on a white tablecloth, just a tiny, still drop of oil, and then in a flash you're expanding outward in every direction, evenly, turning into a stain, a little drop expanding into a bright stain that covers the universe, the process of that, the expanding . . . that's part of it.

Act III—Moreplay: The Return to Balance

After orgasm is the resolution phase, a return to calm and the prearoused state. Men and women differ strikingly in this phase, with the former losing their erections quickly and entering into what's known as a refractory period, an interval of time that needs to pass before he can get an erection again.

With women, it takes longer for the genitals to return to their normal state, at least five to ten minutes. Their genitals don't become hypersensitive (except the clitoral head), and they don't experience a refractory period—with a little stimulation many are ready to begin the process all over again.

The difference between how men and women experience the resolution phase is what I call the "snuggle gap": women want more interaction; men want to roll over and go to sleep. While much literature has been devoted to the "insensitivity" of men and the "neediness" of women in this respect, it's far more effective to understand that the snuggle gap is largely the result of biology (men crash quickly after sex, women come down slowly), so don't overanalyze, or get angry and pick a fight; instead, respect each other's differences and compromise: fall asleep *while* holding her in your arms.

There we have it in a nutshell: the narrative process of arousal. Even though the structure is universal, every story is unique. How it plays out has everything to do with the characters involved. Sometimes the story might unfold in a matter of minutes; other times it may take hours. In the *Poetics*, the only rule is that the action must occur "in a manner uninterrupted," and take place within a twenty-four hour period. As Aristotle observed, "A beautiful object, whether it be a living organism or any whole composed of parts, must not only have an orderly arrangement of parts, but must also be of a certain magnitude; for beauty depends on magnitude and order."

Sounds good to me.

Scent and Sensibility

CUNNILINGUS, perhaps more than any other expression of sexuality, falls prey to the "yes, but" syndrome: YES, both men and women appear on balance to enjoy giving and receiving respectively, BUT not, it seems, without reservation. As noted in the *Hite Report on Male Sexuality*, almost half of all men who said they enjoyed cunnilingus were nonetheless preoccupied with issues of cleanliness and hygiene; and closely associated with those concerns were comments that women's genitals smelled bad. A smaller percentage of men did not share these concerns, and an even smaller group of aficionados claimed to love the taste and smell. But such enthusiasts are in the minority.

Rare is the man who can share Napoleon's steadfast ardor in savoring a woman's *cassolette* (the French word for perfume box and used colloquially to describe a woman's unique scent; the sum total

D on't wash, I'm coming home!" (Napoleon to Josephine, on his way back to Paris from the front.)

of her effluvia; her aromatic signature) and exult, free of prejudice, in the powerful rush of pheromones.

But what about all of the women who—whether bombarded with media messages stressing the importance of feminine "freshness," or worn down by "fish" jokes, or simply unacquainted with their own genitalia—share these preoccupations and approach their bodies with fear, shame, or even self-loathing? And cunnilingus, with its elimination of distance and its unavoidable intimacy, is often a lightning rod for unleashing anxiety.

All this fuss and hullabaloo over hygiene; and yet, in reality, a woman's genitals are a self-cleaning system—*more sanitary than many other parts of the body, including the mouth.* One of the reasons a woman is often lubricated, even when she's not aroused, is that these secretions are part of the vagina's natural way of keeping it bacteria-free. As science writer Natalie Angier has written: "The vagina is its own ecosystem, a land of unsung symbiosis and tart vigor. Sure, the traditional concept of a vagina is 'It's a swamp down there!' but tidal pool would be more accurate: aqueous, stable, yet in perpetual flux."

At the core of this ecosystem is a sophisticated process of symbiosis, one in which healthy bacteria protect and ward off the unhealthy. It's been said that a woman's genitals are as clean as a fresh carton of yogurt, and this comparison is often made because the kind of bacteria found in yogurt, lactobacilli, are also found in a woman's vaginal secretions. In fact, if symbiosis is compromised and unhealthy, anaerobic bacteria gain an advantage, eating yogurt can often help to stave off infection and restore balance.

If there is a bad smell in the genital area, the first thing worth paying attention to is personal hygiene. Like men, women sweat down there and, more often than not, showering or bathing, or even engaging in what the French refer to as a "tart-wash" (a quick freshening of the underarms and genital area) can usually help to rid oneself of any unwanted odors. Later, in Part II, we'll discuss how to eroticize these activities and incorporate hygiene into the excitement.

However, if personal hygiene has been attended to, and an off-putting odor still persists, it's probably time to go to the doctor: she could be suffering from an infection, bacterial vaginosis, in which a lack of lactobacilli creates an imbalance and allows anaerobic bacteria to accumulate. This, according to Natalie Angier, is where the comparison to fish often comes into play, as these microbes produce trimethylamine, the same substance that gives day-old fish its odor.

Gertrude Stein, a cunnilinguist in her own right, may have been mistaken: a rose is a rose is *not always* a rose. Some women are born with imbalances, and might have a predisposition toward vaginosis and a stronger odor. In addition to eating yogurt, there are also antibiotic treatments that can help restore balance.

Every woman smells and tastes different. Some are sweeter than others, some are a bit more pungent, still others are more neutral and nondescript. Sometimes the differences are subtle, other times they're stark. Nor will the same woman always consistently smell or taste the same. Lots of factors can affect smell and taste, including: diet, vitamin deficiencies, medication, her cycle (some women produce vaginal secretions that contain compounds called aliphatic acid chains, and may cause her scent to vary with the phase of her menstrual cycle), infection, hydration, alcohol, drugs, tobacco. Unprotected sex can also affect a woman's smell, in that sperm is highly alkaline and raises the pH level of the vaginal ecosystem.

When it comes to taste and smell, and overall concerns about hygiene, watch out for anxiety brought about by excessive "fear-amone" activity. It's contagious, if not downright viral. Know that a healthy vagina is a clean vagina. Don't let your anxiety trigger a vicious cycle; instead transform that nervous energy into enthusiasm. Enjoy and savor her unique *cassolette*—now there's an idea worth raising a glass to and toasting!

A Question on Scent

Question: "After five years of being monogamous and committed to each other during and after college, my girlfriend and I made a decision to break up in order to see other people. Before we broke up, I had never had any problem with her smell when I went down on her; to be honest I never even noticed it. But then, seven months later, we got back together and I noticed a *distinct* difference. She was more . . . pungent. Eventually her smell returned to normal, but what happened? Could she have had an infection?"

Answer: According to science writer Natalie Angier, a woman can contract vaginosis (an infection that affects her scent) from engaging in unprotected sex. As it turns out, sperm is highly alkaline, more than any other body fluid. When introduced during unprotected sex, this causes the overall pH level of the vagina to rise, and briefly allows unhealthy bacteria to gain advantage.

Usually the body quickly readjusts to normal levels, especially when the sperm is familiar, as it is when two partners are committed to each other and monogamous. But if a woman has unprotected sex with one or more new partners, the body may not be able to restore balance as quickly as possible as a result of immunological factors.

So in some sense, smell may be indicative of promiscuity, and is probably why the *Kamasutra* describes licentious women as smelling like fish.

"In fact, the idea of pairing wine and women isn't a bad one, as the acidity of the vagina in health is just about that of a glass of red wine. This is the vagina that sings; this is the vagina with a bouquet . . ." (Natalie Angier)

Cheers.

We've Come a Long Way . . .

ORAL SEX in America, especially cunnilingus, has come a long, long way.

Back in the 1920s, oral sex (also known as the "genital kiss") was thought to be an activity best left to the marital bed, and was largely deemed a special gesture, a bonus expression of intimacy, but not necessarily a regular part of a couple's sexual practices. It was definitely not a casual activity, and was usually thought to be something that occurred after a couple was already having intercourse in a committed relationship.

So much for the *Roaring* Twenties. Sounds more like the Boring Twenties.

Attitudes began to ease a bit in the 1940s and 1950s, with studies showing that oral sex was becoming more prevalent and better known as a technique that was especially satisfying for women. Even so, in a 1953 *Kinsey Report*, only 3 percent of younger women who were still virgins reported ever receiving cunnilingus. The rate was substantially higher among married women.

During the sexual revolution of the 1960s and 1970s, oral sex evolved into an acceptable practice for *all* couples, whether or not they were married. It became particularly popular on college campuses, and maybe that's why to this day, according to the authors of *Sex in America: A Definitive Survey*, "Twice as many women who went to college have given or received oral sex as compared to those who did not finish high school and twice as many of those better-educated women had or received oral sex the last time they had sex." Finally, the real benefits of a higher education.

Whereas men's rates of receiving oral sex peaked and leveled out in the 1960s, it appears that women spent the remainder of the twentieth century catching up, with rates steadily rising year after year. Today, cunnilingus is considered to be an important part of the arousal process, with enlightened and sexually confident women insisting on quid pro quo—giving according to how they receive. "If there has been any basic change in the script for sex between men and women, it is the increase in the incidence and frequency of fellatio and cunnilingus." (*Sex in America*)

From the conservative to the liberal, women of all stripes enjoy cunnilingus. In examining contemporary sexual mores, the authors of the 1994 *Sex in America Survey* (based on the *National Health and Social Life Survey*) grouped their participants into three different categories: traditional, relational, and recreational.

The traditionalists were those people who maintained that their religious beliefs *always* guided their sexual behavior and believed that homosexuality was wrong; they also believed in restrictions on abortion and did not condone premarital sex, teenage sex, or extramarital sex.

Relationalists believed that sex did not have to be reserved for marriage, but that it should be part of a loving relationship. They condoned premarital sex, but did not condone infidelity or sex without love.

Finally, the recreationalists did not believe that sex need have anything to do with love, and they also opposed laws that prohibited the sale of pornography.

Based on these categories, 83.6 percent of those women with a recreational attitude had experienced oral sex in the last year, followed by 73.9 percent of women who were relational, and 55.9 percent of women with traditional views.

If we look at the numbers in terms of age, 74.7 percent of women from eighteen to twenty-four received oral sex, compared with 73.7 percent of women aged thirty to thirty-four. Women and men aged eighteen to thirty-nine were most likely to include cunnilingus in their sex lives, with 22.3 percent to 24.2 percent reporting having done it during their last sexual experience. Conversely, for women aged forty to forty-four, the rate fell to 12.6 percent. So it would appear that the younger you are the more likely you are to have experienced cunnilingus, and the more likely you are to have experienced it earlier in your lifetime.

As Nancy Friday wrote of cunnilingus in her 1991 book *Women on Top*, "Women have finally come of age. Having discovered it, they can't get enough."

Nor, it seems, can men, for that matter. Happily, this adoption of cunnilingus as a regular part of sexual activity is not just a function of young women becoming more confident and assertive in their demand for a level playing field, but is also indicative of a shift in male attitudes.

As men become more sensitive to the importance of the female orgasm, and recognize the unreliability of genital intercourse in achieving one, they increasingly incorporate cunnilingus into their repertoire of sexual techniques. As *Glamour* magazine noted in their 1997 feature "Good News About Your Sex Life," "A majority of men say they enjoy performing oral sex," and numerous studies report that men describe giving oral sex as very appealing.

If you think it all sounds too good to be true, you're right . . .

18

Eat Right

CUNNILINGUS MAY BE a casual activity, but that doesn't mean you should treat it casually. Make sure that it's part of your safe-sex routine. If you're engaging a new partner, communicate openly and candidly. Be prepared to discuss your current sex partners, sexual history, risky behaviors, STD status, recent activities, and your approach to protection. Be aware that some STDs are asymptomatic and may flourish undetected; so if you find yourself caught up in the heat of the moment, think before engaging in unprotected cunnilingus. Regardless of the reward, even the smallest act is not without risk.

If you're uncertain or nervous, don't take the risk. It's not worth it, and if you don't want to avoid oral sex altogether, then at least take precautions through the use of barriers such as dental dams (a thin strip of latex that is placed over the vulva as you apply cunnilingus), latex gloves, or finger cots (individual plastic sheaths that workers in restaurants use to protect themselves from cuts). All of these safe-sex accessories can typically be found in drugstores, and can also be ordered from specialty stores such as Good Vibrations or the Blowfish catalog. In a pinch, even a sheet of Saran Wrap will do; just make sure you're using the nonmicrowavable kind, as the microwavable sort isn't impervious to bacteria.

If all this talk of protection sounds like a bummer, there is a silver lining: you can definitely have oral sex that is HOT and safe! Later, we will specifically discuss techniques and routines that incorporate safe-sex equipment into the process and do not diminish it. The first step is to know what you need in terms of protection, and then know how to use it.

During sexual activity, a condom is usually not far from reach, and may typically be introduced by either partner. While condoms are generally accepted and prevalent in their use, the same cannot be said of dental dams and the accessories that make for a safe session of cunnilingus. Whereas a request to use a condom is SOP (Standard Operating Procedure) and these days doesn't make one think twice, the introduction of a dental dam is often attention grabbing and may be perceived as signaling the possibility of risk, as opposed to just playing it safe. Perhaps this is because condoms serve the double function of preventing both unwanted pregnancy and unwanted STDs, whereas dental dams only prevent the latter. In short, condoms often embody positive attributes (attentiveness and concern for safety), whereas a dental dam may evoke the negative perception of risk. Rare is the guy who's been carrying a dental dam around in his wallet for years, waiting for the opportunity to put it into use, and equally rare is the woman who's going to insist he use one.

But for all our talk of precaution and protection, there is no substitute for the unfettered merging of our bodies. Like the linking together of two power cables to create a single flow of electricity, your tongue against her vulva is the conjoining of thousands of nerve endings, the firing of neurons, the buzzing of receptors, the ultimate melding of body and soul in a pulse-pounding current. Such joys are ultimately experienced in a trusting, committed relationship. As Sally Tisdale wrote:

> In the depth of sexual passion the skin of the other has the quality of treasure; the mundane secretions our bodies make are honey, manna, light. To be cut off from each other's fluid is a terrible thing; our fluids are meant to mingle, we long for this mingling that is both so outrageous and pure.

When approaching safe sex, keep in mind what Dr. Comfort had to say in *The New Joy of Sex*, "There is no occasion for panic, or for losing out on the joy of sex—simply informed caution."

The Cunnilinguist Manifesto

"From each according to their abilities,
to each according to their needs."
—*The Communist Manifesto*

"To her according to your abilities,
from you according to her needs."
—*The Cunnilinguist Manifesto*

THERE'S NOTHING like strong words to rouse the hearts and minds of men. As we move forward into Part II and focus on specific oral techniques for success, think of Part I as a manifesto, a call to action that urges us first and foremost to:

- Respect the female process of arousal
- Postpone gratification in the pursuit of mutual pleasure
- Know and appreciate the clitoris in all its manifold aspects
- Stimulate the clitoris appropriately through the entire process of sexual response
- Dispense with the conventional wisdom that exalts genital penetration as the apogee of sexual pleasure
- Purge yourself of stereotypes, clichés, and prejudices
- Be patient, respectful, sensitive, and tender

- Take an approach that is pleasure-oriented, not goal-oriented
- Approach each act as a unique process of giving and receiving, knowing and learning
- Give of yourself seriously, generously, and wholeheartedly, even if your relationship is casual and impermanent

Easier said than done. Even Karl Marx recognized that in order for words to become actions, the proper preconditions for success must be firmly in place. In the cunnilinguist revolution, we cannot underestimate the insidious forces of fear, shame, and ignorance.

A woman may be deeply conflicted when it comes to receiving cunnilingus and the experience may be fraught with anxiety. Who knows for sure what emotional baggage she may carry? Take nothing for granted. There's an utter nakedness to cunnilingus, a vulnerability that we must respect and honor. She is exposing herself to be seen, smelled, tasted, and observed firsthand; she is permitting the exploration of a part of her body that she herself may find unfamiliar and mysterious. She may think her vulva is ugly, unkempt, unpredictable in its secretions, odoriferous, and strange. She may insist on making love in the dark, literally and figuratively.

A cunnilinguist needs to be committed, steadfast, and confident in his resolve. If she senses that he's the least bit ambivalent, insincere, or impatient, then his efforts will be for naught. Only by inspiring trust will you lull her into a deeper, more instinctive zone of the self, a place where she can shed all inhibition and surrender herself to the soft warm wetness of your tongue.

To that end, the Three Assurances of the cunnilinguist manifesto are as follows:

- Going down on her turns *you* on; you enjoy it as much as she does.
- There's no rush; she has all the time in the world. You want to savor every moment.

- Her scent is provocative, her taste powerful: it all emanates from the same beautiful essence.

Communicate these Three Assurances physically and verbally; repeat them over and over, in every possible way; say them, show them: embody them. Be strong, be understanding. If she has issues, fears, talk your way through them. Work your way through the anxiety. Lead her to a breakthrough. Be one of the good guys.

Take one small lick for man, one giant lick for womankind.

Cunnilinguists of the world unite. The revolution is upon us.

Vive la Vulva!

PART

Rules of Usage

TWO

"Here is a perfect poem:
to awaken a longing, to nourish it,
to develop it, to increase it, to stimulate it—and
to gratify it."

—Balzac

A Note on the Play Process

AS DISCUSSED IN PART I, cunnilingus has been tradition-ally considered an optional aspect of foreplay rather than a sexual act in its own right that can lead a woman through the entire process of sexual response.

In relegating oral sex (as well as other important activities such as manual stimulation of the clitoris) to the domain of foreplay we are simultaneously:

- Discounting the importance of these pleasure-oriented activities
- Limiting their role in the overall process of arousal/sexual response
- Promoting genital penetration as the centerpiece of sexual experience

In doing so, we open a chasm between tongue and clitoris—one that often cannot be bridged by the penis.

Additionally, the relegation of cunnilingus to foreplay reinforces the false idea that the tongue is best applied during the early stages of sexual response, when in fact the opposite is true: because of the heightened sensitivity of the clitoris, direct stimulation is best approached slowly and gradually, and is ideally preceded by a variety of erotic activities.

In short, cunnilingus is *not* foreplay, it's *coreplay*, the best approach for consistently applying various methods of clitoral stimulation; and one that, like genital penetration, requires an appropriate prologue of erotic activity. Hence, in our discussion of technique, *foreplay* will be considered those activities that precede coreplay—the sublime waltz of tongue and clitoris.

As Aristotle noted, "A middle is only a middle when preceded by a beginning and followed by an end." Whereas for men, the completion of the process of sexual response virtually converges with the explosion of orgasm, it has been amply demonstrated that a woman, upon climaxing, requires a greater period of time to return to the prearoused state; hence, the importance of *moreplay*.

And so there we have it, the play process: foreplay, coreplay, and moreplay—taken as a whole, the makings of great sexual drama.

Time to put on a show.

Foreplay: A Lexicon of Relevant Terms

"A bad beginning makes a bad ending."
—Euripides

"Do not take shortcuts at the cost of clarity."
—*Elements of Style*

Anticipation: Create a strong sense of expectation. A little goes a long way: a hot, hushed phone call from work, a furtive whisper over dinner, a glancing touch on the nape of the neck. The smallest of gestures can imbue the banal with erotic energy and electrify the mundane.

Avoid: During foreplay avoid direct contact with her genitals for a minimum of ten to fifteen minutes. Stimulate other parts of her body; let the oxytocin wash over her. Save the genital kiss for last, as the first kiss upon the vulva is the threshold between foreplay and coreplay.

Awareness: Stay attuned to the nuances of sexual response; don't lose your focus, or let the process slip away from you. Every moment builds continuously on the last to create a seamless experience. Remember what Aristotle said, "Most important of all is the structure of the incidents. If any one of them is displaced or removed, the whole will be disjointed and disturbed."

Bath, a: Cleanliness is an important part of any sexual encounter, but particularly in respect to cunnilingus. Squeamishness regarding genital hygiene is the number one reservation that men level against cunnilingus, and is also a source of anxiety for women who worry that their partners may be wary. Incorporate a shared bath or shower into foreplay. Channel the anxiety into a romantic event.

Beard: Unless you have a full, soft beard, consider shaving, as stubble can irritate her vulva, inner thighs, and other sensitive areas.

Body, hers: Keep in mind that skin is our largest sexual organ, and the entire body, from head to toe, is one big erogenous zone. This is especially true of women, as the female body is generally smaller than the male and the same numbers of nerves are consequently dispersed across a smaller surface area; hence the number of sensitive receptors is proportionally larger on the female body. Second, the female skin is generally thinner and less hairy than the male, so sensations are more clearly felt. Sex researchers have observed that some women can reach orgasm by simply having their eyebrows stroked or their earlobes kissed. As Voltaire wrote, "Love is a canvas furnished by Nature and embroidered by imagination."

Breasts: While there is indeed a biological basis for the pleasure connection between breasts and vulva in the form of oxytocin—a chemical that heightens our sensitivity to touch and is released in her genital area when the breasts are stimulated—numerous studies reveal that breast contact often stimulates *men* more than it does women. In a Kinsey study of female sexual response, only 11 percent of the eight thousand women surveyed said that they stroked their breasts during masturbation (compared to 84 percent who stroked their clitoris or labia minora). So it stands to reason that when it comes to her breasts, a significant component of her pleasure is the enjoyment of yours. Every woman is different regarding the breast sensitivity, so err on the side of tenderness and look for feedback. As one of this author's interviewees put it, "Savor, don't suckle."

Breath, bad: In all this fuss about hygiene, don't forget about your own, particularly oral, as there are more bacteria in the mouth than in the vagina. Rather than brushing your teeth, which could cause cuts and sores and raise the risk of spreading or contracting an STD, simply rinse well with a *mild* mouthwash. Stay away from floss prior to sexual activity for the same reasons.

Breathing, hers: Most men think of vaginal wetness as the most reliable indicator of a woman's level of arousal; and while there is indeed a strong correlation between lubrication and sexual response, she may or may not be wet for reasons that have nothing to do with her level of sexual excitement. Breathing, on the other hand, is an oft-neglected indicator. As she gets more aroused, look for the commensurate changes in her breathing, and tightening of the abdominal muscles.

Candles: Men and women differ when it comes to their attitudes about doing it with the lights on. Like Hemingway, men often enjoy "a clean, well-lighted place" in which to practice and observe their craft, whereas women often prefer the cover of dark. Compromise with candlelight.

Communication: Keep all channels open throughout the process, verbal and physical; maintain a persistent feedback loop of stimulation and response. According to *Sex: A Man's Guide,* "In a *Redbook* magazine survey of 100,000 married women, the strongest indicator of sexual and marital satisfaction among them was the ability to express sexual feelings to their husbands. The more they talked, the better they rated their sex lives, their marriages and their overall happiness." Let each other know what works, as well as what doesn't. Be positive and constructive; *criticism, expressed harshly, is often the death of sex.*

Fantasies: So potent is the power of the imagination that some women are actually able to fantasize themselves to orgasm, without any physical stimulation at all. Studies reveal that men and women fantasize differently. In general, women tend to fantasize in ways that are more situational and narrative, whereas men's fantasies tend to focus more on specific physical and graphical elements of sexual encounters.

In terms of subject matter, there is overlap between men and women, with common fantasies including: multiple partners, soft bondage, anal play, cheating, watching others voyeuristically, and having sex in public places, among many others.

Fantasize, together: Take a page from *The Thousand and One Nights* and incorporate a story into foreplay. If you're not a born storyteller, try reading one aloud together. Some literary recommendations: James Salter's erotic masterpiece, *A Sport and a Pastime*; Anais Nin's collections of short stories *Delta of Venus* and *Little Birds*; the erotic novels *Emanuelle* by Emanuelle Arsan and *Story of O* by Pauline Réage; Harold Brodkey's sexual saga "Innocence"— perhaps the greatest depiction of a session of cunnilingus ever penned; novels by Jerzy Kosinski such as *Passion Play* and *Cockpit*; Henry Miller's *Under the Roofs of Paris* and *Quiet Days in Clichy*; *My Secret Life* by Anonymous and *The Pure and the Impure* by Colette; Nancy Friday's anthology of fantasies, *Secret Garden* (filled with the correspondence of real people's fantasies); stories from *The Mammoth Book of Erotica* or one of the many erotic anthologies edited by Susie Bright. For those with a taste for poetry, try *Les Fleurs du Mal* (Flowers of Evil) by Charles Baudelaire or *Flesh Unlimited* by Guillaume Apollinaire. And for those who like comic books (kinky ones, that is), try the extra-hot works of writer/illustrator Eric Stanton, who specializes in female-domination fantasies.

Fantasize, separately: Keep in mind that there are those fantasies we share aloud, and others we keep to ourselves. Respect each other's privacy, and don't be threatened by what's in her imagination. According to the authors of *Sex: A Man's Guide*, studies reveal that about 85 percent of both men and women have sexual fantasies during sexual intercourse some of the time. The authors go on to cite a study by Harold Leitenberg, Ph.D., in which he concludes that people who fantasize during sex feel a greater level of sexual satisfaction and have fewer sexual problems in their relationships—

even if the person about whom they fantasize is *different* from the person they have a relationship with.

"At times I find it's harder to talk about my fantasies than my actual sexual experience. What I *do* sexually is the product of many factors, not all of them sexually motivated. But what I *imagine* doing is pure—pure in the sense that the image comes wholly from within, from the soil of the subconscious. The land of the fantasy is the land of the not-done and wished for." (Tisdale)

Fantasy vs. Reality: Note the difference between sharing a fantasy and acting one out. The former is harmless and exploratory; the latter can often lead to unforeseen consequences unless discussed and properly understood by everyone concerned. This is even truer when a fantasy is taken out of the bedroom. The sex we have in our lives—familiar, repetitious—is usually very different from the sex we have in our fantasies—exaggerated, taboo—and perhaps that's the point. Think twice before taking fantasies out of the bedroom, and know that a rich inner life contributes to a healthy, happy outer one. As one interviewee commented, "Even if I wanted to live out my fantasies, it's impossible. I'd need a time machine *and* a spaceship."

Fellatio: One of her greatest sources of pleasure will be to pleasure you, and there's no better way for her to do so than with some generous oral attention. Just don't get too carried away. Numerous surveys note that men enjoy fellatio as much as, if not more than, intercourse, and that it's the easiest way for a woman to stimulate a man to orgasm. Receiving head is not permission to ejaculate. As Dr. Comfort wrote in *The New Joy of Sex*, "A few men can't take even the shortest genital kiss before ejaculating." So if fellatio is something you love and must have, then go for a "light snack" during foreplay and put in your request for prolonged attention after coreplay.

Fingers, stimulation: Once she's aroused—her body awoken and sensitized by your attention—manual stimulation of her vulva will prove to be the pièce de résistance of foreplay; plan on taking ample time to deploy just the right combination of pressure, motion, and rhythm.

Before you get going, you might want to moisten your hands with some lubricant (see *Lubricant* for the ins and outs of choosing the right one), although at this point her natural lubrication should be in steady flow. Also, make sure your fingernails are clipped, as they can irritate her genital area, as well as cause small scratches and cuts. For step-by-step instructions and illustrations on how to use your fingers like a virtuoso, see the Appendix.

Hair, pubic: When it comes to hair care, guys care. Some men love it and can't get enough of it; all they want to do is rub their noses in it and take in the full aroma of a woman's scent. Others prefer a neatly trimmed coif; still others enjoy the thin strip of a Mohawk or the sleek, bald pate of a naked vulva—what the Chinese refer to as "the White Tiger." Ultimately, it's her decision. Remember that; respect it. Some women don't want the hassle of having to attend to *yet another* aspect of their appearance, and anything beyond a mild trim is going to involve discomfort, itching, and perhaps even pain.

Kissing: As Shelley wrote, "Soul meets soul on lovers' lips." A kiss is like the contact of two chemical substances: if there is any reaction, both are transformed. A kiss is a unique and versatile expression of the soul. A kiss can be playful, patient, and coy; or ravenous, forceful, and violent. According to the teachings of Tantra, a woman's upper lip is considered one of the most erogenous areas on her body because of a special nerve that connects it to the clitoris, and is said to channel erotic energy. Like language itself, there is virtually no emotion that cannot be expressed with a kiss. *Cunnilingus is simply the art of extending a kiss into a complete act of lovemaking.*

Language: "All the fun's in how you say a thing," wrote Robert Frost, and this couldn't be truer than when applied to sex play. According to a survey in *Men's Fitness* magazine, over 90 percent of men love it when their partners talk dirty to them. So if you tend to be the quiet type in bed, untie your tongue and verbalize your erotic feelings.

But pick your words wisely, and remember what Mark Twain had to say in this regard: "The difference between the right word and the nearly right word is the same as that between lightning and the lightning bug." The same is true of "turnoff" and "turn-on," so make sure your choice of words has the latter effect, not the former.

When searching for the right words, remember what *Elements of Style* had to say, "All writers, by the way they use language, reveal something of their spirits, their habits, their capacities and their biases."

Lingerie: Appreciate before proceeding to rip, tear, and ravish. Unlike guys, whose capacity for creativity in the area of underwear selection rarely extends beyond deciding between boxers or briefs, women often apply considerable resources—physical, creative, financial—in order to be well diversified in this department. As one interviewee commented, "Who the hell does he think he is, Conan the Barbarian? He tore through my panties with his teeth. Excuse me, but those were fifty-dollar La Perla!"

Lubricant, artificial: There's an old Malagasy proverb, "Let your love be like the misty rain, coming softly, but flooding the river." But if your partner doesn't lubricate consistently, easily, or at all, don't take it personally. In a 1994 *Sex in America Survey,* 20 percent of women complained of trouble lubricating when engaging in sexual activity.

In terms of cunnilingus, artificial lubricant is neither as important nor as indispensable as it is during genital intercourse. As Dr. Comfort noted in *The New Joy of Sex,* "The best sexual lubricant is saliva" and it's usually in ample supply during cunnilingus. But even the mouth grows dry at times, so it never hurts to have some water-based lubricant close at hand.

In selecting a lubricant, read the ingredients carefully and stay away from those that are oil-based and contain chemicals such as nonoxynol-9, a commonly used spermicidal that tastes awful, and can burn and lead to infection. Also, stay away from jellies, such as K-Y, that are greasy and heavy. Best to choose a water-based product that has few ingredients. Astroglide is a common favorite, and has earned the reputation of its tagline, "second only to nature." There's no shortage of choices, so enjoy the process of selection.

Massage, foot: One of the most underestimated and underutilized forms of erotic stimulation, a good solid foot massage floods the bloodstream with endorphins and energizes the entire body. No need to worry about not being a professional masseur, just maintain persistent contact between hand and foot, massaging one foot at a time with both hands. Work the whole foot: the sole, ball, ankle, and toe joints before going to the other one. Feel free to kiss her toes. Some women won't be able to stand it, while others will experience the heights of pleasure.

Masturbation: Sex researchers Masters and Johnson gathered much of their information about female sexual response by watching women masturbate. Take note: they consistently observed that women focused their manual stimulation on the clitoral head, as well as the shaft, mons pubis, and inner and outer labia. Because of the heightened sensitivity of the head, most women stimulated it at the peak of arousal, and avoided direct contact immediately subsequent to orgasm. Dr. Kinsey found that 95 percent of the women he studied climaxed far more often through masturbation than during genital penetration. This observation was corroborated by Masters and Johnson, who found that over 90 percent of women were able to experience an orgasm through masturbation.

Although Masters and Johnson observed consistencies in how women masturbated, they also emphasized that no two women masturbated in exactly the same way.

Masturbation, shared: Not necessarily for her eyes only, but an opportunity to observe a woman's unique way of consistently bringing herself to climax—something clearly worth studying. But remember: even though masturbation is a common, often shared experience, it's still as close to taboo as you can get these days. In his book *Solitary Sex: A Cultural History of Masturbation*, Thomas Laqueur, a history professor at the University of California, Berkeley, writes, "In general, masturbation is that rare thing in modern talk about sexuality: something best left unspoken and so discomfiting that it can only be broached as a joke."

If she's never masturbated in front of you, create an environment of intimacy and trust. Most important, let her know that it's something you want her to do because it turns you on and because you want to learn more about how to please her.

Regardless of the hurdles, it will improve your sex life when you are comfortable sharing the act of masturbation with each other. It will not only prove erotically stimulating, but masturbation will also serve as a reliable fallback for those times when, for one reason or another, sexual activity does not lead her to orgasm and she needs to take matters into her own hands.

Music: Use it to enhance the mood, not kill it. Find music that lulls you *both* into a deeper zone of letting go, music that helps you synchronize yourselves into a mutual sense of rhythm and pacing. The right choice can really stimulate the senses; the wrong choice can shut them down. One interviewee commented that she likes to play Ravel's *Boléro* during sex as "it both captures and stimulates the process of arousal—the way the tension builds slowly, repetitiously . . . subliminally encouraging my boyfriend to slow down and wait until it all builds to a crescendo." Yet another woman commented, "This may sound weird, but I love to listen to whale music when a guy goes down on me. I have all these bizarre underwater fantasies. Sometimes I even imagine that I'm the female whale and that I'm being called by the male whale, with his like, what, fifty-foot cock."

Orgasms, multiple: Oftentimes a woman will experience an orgasm during foreplay, particularly if ample stimulation has been effectively applied. While all women have the innate biological capacity for multiple orgasms, not all have experienced them and many might be unaware of their inherent potential. If she experiences one during foreplay, transition for a few minutes into a milder form of stimulation such as kissing and hugging before moving into coreplay. This shift in activity is particularly essential if her orgasm was the result of manual stimulation of the clitoris, as the clitoral head is particularly sensitive to touch following orgasm. Let her cool down, but keep her warm and sexualized by focusing your attention on other parts of her body. After this brief interval, you will be able to return to direct stimulation of her vulva and get ready for her next orgasm.

Penetration: If cunnilingus is coreplay, then it's possible to think of genital penetration as an aspect of part of foreplay. In the standard missionary position—you on top, her beneath you—use the tip of your penis to barely penetrate her vaginal entrance. Let your penis rest just inside her. (If you're uncomfortable in the missionary position, then simply kneel or sit in front of her vulva.) Linger. Loiter. Meander. Stay close to the entrance. Press your thumb against her clitoral head and gently flick it from side to side as you penetrate her with short shallow thrusts. Or press the shaft of your penis against her clitoris and then gently thrust between the folds of her labia without ever entering her. Or she can perform Kegels (the squeezing of her pelvic muscles) while you, ever so slowly, penetrate her. Really take the time to feel her pelvic muscles contract against your penis as you slowly withdraw.

Style: Don't be a show-off. As written in *Elements of Style*, "The beginner should approach style warily, realizing that it is an expression of self, and should turn resolutely away from all devices that are popularly believed to indicate style—all mannerisms, tricks, adornments. The approach to style is by way of plainness, simplicity, orderliness, sincerity."

Holds true for experts as well.

Ties: The kind that bind. Restraining a lover during sexual activity is a popular fantasy, and one that, unlike some others, is easily realized, and erotically rewarding. When approached safely as a light-hearted, playful activity, restraint is a fun, guilt-free way of acting out dominance roles and expressing healthy sexual aggression. It stimulates her body by allowing her to flex her muscles more intensely than when unrestrained; it also stimulates her mind by allowing her to surrender to pleasure and act out in ways that might normally make her feel awkward or shy. It also encourages you to take your time and lavish her with attention as she submits to your teasing. From constraint comes creativity. If you're new to this topic, err on the side of caution and peruse the pointers in the Appendix before proceeding.

Time: Take lots of it. As Ovid wrote, "Love's climax should never be rushed I say / But worked up slowly, lingering all the way."

Introducing Coreplay

"Proper words in their proper place make
the true definition of a style."
—Jonathan Swift

ALTHOUGH IT'S IMPERATIVE that the play process unfold
seamlessly from beginning to end, without interruption, it is
nonetheless useful, in discussion, to break the process down into
substages, especially as they help to illuminate coreplay—the sub-
stantive phase in which sexual tension builds, culminates, and then
releases itself through the female orgasm.

Therefore, we will discuss coreplay in terms of six distinct stages
that are easy to understand:

- **Stage 1:** in which we transition from foreplay to coreplay
with the application of the first clitoral kiss
- **Stage 2:** in which we establish rhythm and acclimate the
clitoris to the persistent attentions of the tongue
- **Stage 3:** in which we continue to build tension by focusing

more of our energies on the clitoral head, as well as introducing appropriate manual stimulation

- **Stage 4:** in which we hypercharge the process of sexual response and escalate her level of arousal by internally stimulating the "clitoral cluster" in combination with the clitoral head
- **Stage 5:** preorgasm, in which we maintain the optimum balance of rhythm and pressure as she approaches orgasm
- **Stage 6:** Orgasm, in which we maximize the number of pelvic contractions and help her to realize the full potential of her climax

In abbreviated terms, think of these stages as a straightforward process that encompasses: the first kiss; establishing rhythm; building tension; escalating the action; preorgasm and orgasm.

Going forward, we will dedicate our attention to a more thorough discussion of these six substages of coreplay, explore related topics that arise throughout the process of female sexual response, and break down an array of techniques that will keep the action going.

But first, before we do anything, let's make sure we're in the right position . . .

Form Follows Function: Getting into Position

BEFORE GOING DOWN on a woman, make sure to position yourself for maximum performance. Bad form is often the difference between success and failure. Porn films would have us believe that *any* position is the right position: up against the wall, on top of a table, hanging off the bed, hanging off the rafters—the wilder the better. But it should come as no surprise that with titles like *Hannah Does Her Sisters* or *Titty Titty Bang Bang*, the porn industry, in general, shies away from the lofty aesthetics of cinema vérité.

First and foremost, expert cunnilingus needs to be delivered from a position that enables the giver to *comfortably* apply persistent, rhythmic pressure over time while the receiver relaxes into the nuances of arousal. Not surprisingly, one of the main reasons why men say they don't perform cunnilingus more often is the physical strain—in short, the pain of being in the wrong position. So if your attitude toward cunnilingus is "no pain, no gain," the sentiment is appreciated, but entirely unnecessary.

First, the Wrong Way

There are a few positions, better suited to porn films than to prolonged clitoral stimulation, that have nonetheless become widely, and wrongy, disseminated into the mainstream. At best they serve as spicy embellishments to a session of cunnilingus; at worst they can seriously undermine the entire experience. These popular positions include 69'ing, SOMF (Sit on My Face), and Up Against the Wall, among others.

69'ing

Of the three positions mentioned, 69'ing, in which man and woman service each other simultaneously, is probably the most prevalent and also the most problematic:

- In the 69 position, you are endeavoring to provide stimulation from the wrong orientation. Rather than approaching her vulva from the south (bottom up), you're coming in from the north (top down). Regardless of who's on top, you'll have little use of your hands and it will be difficult to use your tongue to comfortably service the major parts of her clitoris. As author and sex columnist Anka Radakovich writes of the position: "Working out the logistics of fitting mouths on orifices and protrusions while adjusting to the rhythm is like playing a game of Naked Twister."
- If you're giving while simultaneously receiving, it's highly unlikely that you'll be able to focus on the application of measured, evenhanded clitoral stimulation There's even a

chance that you'll get caught up in the moment and allow yourself to lose control.

- Finally, the position cannot be comfortably sustained at length, nor can she fully relax and concentrate on the nuances of arousal. The fact is, when it comes to oral sex, it's best for one partner to focus on giving while the other focuses on receiving.

In short, 69'ing is a novelty act. That's not to say it isn't an exciting position, or a compelling means of enabling her to enjoy the pleasure of pleasuring you, but such joys are best experienced during foreplay—not coreplay.

When 69'ing during foreplay, make sure you don't waste your best tongue strokes: save them for coreplay. The first kiss upon her vulva should take her breath away, so don't diminish the sense of anticipation. Instead, kiss the areas *around* the vulva rather than the clitoris. Use your lips, not your tongue. Smooch. Nibble. But stay away from the clitoral head. Turn the position into one of strength; use it as a way of teasing her to greater heights.

SOMF (Sit on My Face)

The same can be said of SOMF, a position that provides you with better access to her vulva than 69'ing but significantly hinders the use of your hands and fingers—a trade-off without much real gain. Sitting on your face (really kneeling *around* your face) forces her into an upright position and places undue stress on her back and legs. In this position, it's highly unlikely she'll get very far in the process of sexual response; however, it can prove erotically stimulating by providing her with a sense of dominance, and might be good for a bit of fun.

Up Against the Wall

In Up Against the Wall she literally stands against a wall while you kneel down before her. Although it's unlikely that she'll reach orgasm from this position, with a wall to provide support it's easier to lead her through several stages of arousal. Up Against the Wall has all the rough passion of a "quickie," but without the male ejaculation that often accompanies the genital version of this position.

All three of these positions—69'ing, SOMF, and Up Against the Wall—are useful in that they provide erotic stimulation and often heighten the drama of the moment. In fact, with a little help from your imagination, there's no limit to the number of creative positions that can be devised and put to the test—one book I came across actually recommends going down on a woman while she stands on her head with her legs wrapped around your neck. Use these positions during foreplay to accelerate the process of arousal into coreplay, but don't mistake them for the ones that enable the application of *serious* clitoral stimulation to the point of no return.

So much for the wrong way . . .

Now the Right Way

Her Body

- She should start flat on her back, legs spread comfortably apart, but not too far (six to nine inches at most) and a bit bent at the knee. As a rule, her legs should always be closer together than farther apart, as she needs the full command of her pelvic muscles. She should be completely at ease and relaxed: able to focus on the pleasure she's receiving without any distraction—physical or mental.
- Pay attention to the arch of her back. Once again, we get the idea from porn that when a woman is turned on she

naturally arches her back upward, throws back her head, and points her breasts and neck up and out. This position, while titillating, is what the famous sexologist Wilhelm Reich referred to as the "hysterical arch." Not only is it highly unnatural, but the position also cuts off blood flow to the pelvic area, hampers breathing, and inhibits the process of sexual response. When a woman is aroused and comfortable, her back will find itself flat, without an arch, and her genitals will be tilted slightly up toward your mouth, rather than driving downward—in short, the opposite of what we see in porn. To help her achieve this naturally comfortable position, prop a pillow or two behind her neck and shoulders.

A pillow propped under her butt will help with blood flow to the pelvic region, as well as provide you with better access to her genitalia, making it easier for you to connect "lips" and alleviate stress to your neck.

Your Body

It's important that you have enough space to stretch out and be comfortable—so you'll probably have to push her up toward the head of the bed. (If you're both on the floor—also a great place for a session of cunnilingus in that the floor provides a solid flat surface—just make sure there's some sort of cushioning beneath her, be it a soft rug or plush quilt.)

- Place a pillow beneath your forearms and get your "working hands" as comfortable and close as possible to her vulva.
- Position yourself vertically from her vagina. Other than the *narrow* flaring of her legs, your bodies, taken together, should form a straight line.
- All in all, you should feel perfectly at ease adopting a wide range of motions: licking for long periods of time, sliding

If you grapple with a form of sexual dysfunction, namely premature ejaculation or erectile disorder (also known as impotence), go to the Appendix, where you'll find specific body positions geared to help you turn your weaknesses into strengths.

your hands underneath her butt, lifting her legs and rocking her to and fro, placing a hand on her stomach, turning her body from side to side.

Your Head

- They don't call it "giving head" for nothing. Cunnilingus involves more than just the use of your tongue. You need to get your whole face in there. Your nose should be buried lightly in her mound, with your upper lip and mustache area resting firmly against the front edge of her pubic bone. You should be able to easily use your upper lip and gum to provide light pressure against her front commissure, the area just above the clitoral head where her outer lips meet.
- As for your tongue, it should easily be able to rest against her vaginal entrance and cover its entire expanse from top to bottom. This position enables you to apply a full range of motion with your tongue: from long vigorous licks to deft persistent flicks, from keeping it flat and still to applying focused tongue-tip pressure.
- All in all, you should be completely involved with her vulva; on top of it, buried in it: face, mouth, nose, gums, teeth, and tongue—all of which will be employed one way or another. If a filmmaker were capturing the event, very little would be seen beyond the still back of your head. Certainly, there would be few, if any, flashes of tongue.

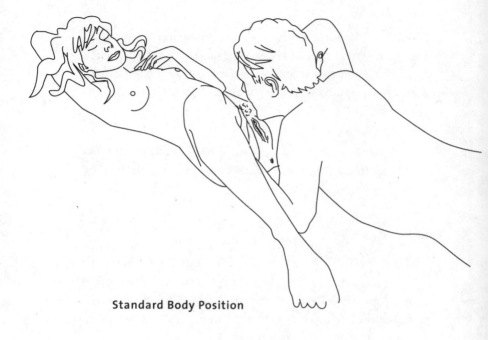

Standard Body Position

Taken Together

Don't settle for anything less than total comfort and total access. You'll know you're both in the right position when she's able to comfortably look down the length of her body and watch you work, and you're able to look up, without breaking the flow of action, and make eye contact with her.

When it comes to cunnilingus and body position, remember that form *follows* function. Keep your mind focused on providing her with pleasure, and the body will naturally follow your lead.

Head Position

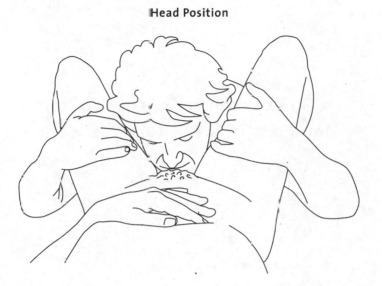

Let's Review

In this chapter we discussed the importance of getting off to a good start by being in the right position. Make sure you're comfortable and relaxed. Avoid novelty positions that restrict the use of your hands and fingers and might also cut off the flow of blood to her pelvic area or inhibit the process of sexual response. Find positions that enable you to optimally exploit your respective roles of giver and receiver.

A Quick Refresher of the Top Ten
Hot Spots in the Clitoral Network

A S WE VEER into coreplay, let's quickly review the areas of the clitoral network that are going to command our attention, as well as the types of stimulation to which they're best suited. (This is a great time to refer back to the diagrams of the clitoral network in Part I and use them as a visual reference.) Don't get overwhelmed by the numerous the parts of the clitoris. It may seem like a lot to take in at first, but a little effort goes a long, *long* way. Trust me: as we go through the various techniques, the "geography of arousal" will become second nature and you'll know a "frenulum" from a "front commissure" in no time. And take heart: simply knowing "what's what" in the clitoral network *already* places you at the head of the class.

1. Glans (visible), also known as the head or crown and colloquially as the clit, the button, the jewel, etc. With more than eight thousand nerve endings dedicated to pleasure, the glans lends truth to the phrase "big things come in small packages." So sensitive is the glans to stimulation that a *hood*, also known as the prepuce, protects it during peak stimulation. Both the clitoral head and its protective hood respond to gentle, rhythmic tongue strokes as well as firmer pressure once she's well into the process of arousal.

2. Clitoral cluster (hidden) includes what is typically referred to as the G-spot, but to call this sensitive expanse a spot is a misnomer. Located atop the vaginal ceiling—starting at the vaginal entrance and extending into the birth canal for roughly two inches—this area of spongy tissue surrounds the urethra and responds well to the firm pressure of a fingertip massage. Rather than focus on finding a spot, focus on stimulating an area.

3. Mons pubis (external), or the pubic mound, is located just above the clitoral cluster. Massaging the mons pubis with the base of your palm stimulates the clitoral cluster from above. Think of the clitoral cluster as an unseen layer of nerve endings that is sandwiched between the mons pubis and the vaginal canal—hence your ability to stimulate it from above and below.

4. Front commissure (external). The smooth area just above the clitoral head and protective hood, this area contains nerve fibers and covers the *clitoral shaft* (internal), a sensitive cordlike structure that can be seen protruding from the skin of the front commissure when aroused. Like the clitoral head, the front commissure/shaft responds at first to tongue strokes, but, once aroused, craves the firmer pressure of the upper lip and gum, or a fingertip massage.

5. Frenulum (external) is the area just below the clitoral head where the tops of labia minora (the inner lips) meet. This sensitive area responds to tongue strokes as well as firm pressure. Like the glans and

A "Sensitive" Question

Question: "My girlfriend says she doesn't like cunnilingus because it hurts. I don't get it. How can it hurt? I went down on her once and now she won't let me do it again. What did I do wrong?" (Steve, 32)

Answer: You may have been too rough, or overzealous, without even realizing it. Ask her if you can try again, and assure her that this time you'll be gentle. Let her know that you'll stop immediately if she says the word. Remember that the glans is extremely sensitive, and many women cannot bear even the slightest contact—particularly at the start of a cunnilingus session.

Going forward, be as gentle as possible and avoid direct contact with the head until she's amply aroused. Focus on her labia and vaginal entrance; pay attention to her perineum. Don't forget about her front commissure and frenulum, the area just above and below the head. Apply halfway licks instead of full licks, avoid the head completely.

When you do stimulate the head for the first time, press the soft, wet tip of your tongue into it and then hold the position. Like a gentle mist, engulf the head in the moistness of your tongue. She might shudder from the shock, but continue to hold the position unless she tells you to stop.

Let her ease into the feeling of your tongue against her clitoris. Stay still, let her initiate the movement; let her determine the appropriate amount of pressure to apply against your tongue. Let her lead in the dance between clitoris and tongue.

front commissure/shaft, the frenulum plays an important role in sexual response. In fact, taken together, these three visible parts of the clitoris are responsible for the lion's share of pleasure.

6. Labia minora (external), also known as the little lips or the inner lips, they swell to nearly double their size when engorged with blood during arousal and respond best to tongue strokes, gentle nibbles, and playful fingertip pinches.

7. Vaginal entrance (external) contains the remnants of the hymen and, when amply aroused and lubricated, responds best to slow, long licks and gentle fingertip tickles.

8. Fourchette (external) is the area located at the base of the vaginal entrance where the bottoms of the labia minora converge, and responds best to tongue strokes and gentle fingertip tickles that just graze the vaginal entrance.

9. Perineum (external) is the expanse of skin between the fourchette and anus and is filled with spongy erectile tissue that connects the anus to the clitoral network and lines the base of the vagina. This area responds well to tongue strokes, fingertip pressure, and fingertip squeezes (thumb and index finger) that stimulate it from both sides (internal and external).

10. Anus (external). Lined with tissue and muscle that connects it to the clitoral network, the anus participates in the process of sexual response and, like the pelvic muscles, contracts repeatedly during orgasm. This area responds well to fingertip pressure, fingertip insertion, and tongue strokes, but also contains bacteria that should be prevented from commingling with other parts of the vulva.

Grand Openings:
The First Kiss

The Approach

NEVER UNDERESTIMATE the power of first impressions, especially the impression of your lips against her vulva. The first kiss atop a woman's vulva is often the most exquisite of all possible kisses and can literally take her breath away.

Approach the first kiss as an event, as though tasting the first sip of an expensive bottle of wine that you've been saving for that special occasion. Don't just pop off the cork and start swigging: let it breathe, sniff and savor the bouquet, admire the body, note the complexion and tone, and then, finally, take that much anticipated first sip. Allow yourself to appreciate the full experience.

- Run your fingers gently through her pubic hair.
- Be sure to tease her amply. Kiss her softly on the inner thigh,

as well as the smooth skin adjoining her vulva. Kiss her with little, succulent smacks (lips pursed, no tongue) on her inner and outer lips, or even on the top of the head. Make sure that your first kiss is less about direct contact with the clitoris and more about appreciating the entire genital area.

- Breathe hotly on her vulva.
- Blow, ever so gently, *on* her clitoral head.
- If she's still wearing her panties, kiss her *through* them. Then delicately peel them to the side to reveal a glistening wet vulva.

CAUTION: Never, under *any* circumstances, blow *into* a woman's vagina as though trying to fill it with air. Doing so is *seriously* dangerous. Blowing into a woman's vagina may cause an embolism and lead to death. Breathe *on* her; blow lightly *on* her; *never* blow *into* her.

The Moment Before

Before you move in for the first kiss, take a moment to acknowledge the presence of the vulva: your partner in pleasure. Prepare yourself mentally for the experience ahead. Remind yourself that you are there to join her steadfastly through the process of sexual response to orgasm.

This is a great time to remind her of the Three Assurances (see part I, chapter 20):

- Going down on her turns *you* on; you enjoy it as much as she does.
- There's no rush; she has all the time in the world. You want to savor every moment.
- Her scent is provocative, her taste powerful: it all emanates from the same beautiful essence.

Like a guest arriving at a much-anticipated dinner party, let your hostess know how excited you are to be there, how beautiful she looks, and how much you're looking forward to the meal ahead. Put her at ease.

Tease her, taunt her, tantalize her—make her think that she's not ever going to get it, *ever*, and then, just when she's on the brink of utter madness, give it to her.

The Kiss

Make your first lick a slow and tender "ice cream" lick from bottom to top. Make it long and lasting. Take it all in.

- Start at the base of her vaginal entrance, the fourchette, and work your way up.
- Take in the full length of her labia minora (inner lips) and let your tongue rest briefly against her frenulum, the area just under the clitoral head.
- As you go over the head, brush it lightly as a feather, and then proceed to her front commissure (the area just above the head).
- Push down on her commissure with the tip of your tongue and feel the sinewy clitoral shaft beneath it.
- As you kiss her slowly from top to bottom, press your finger lightly against her perineum (the expanse of skin just below her vaginal entrance).
- When you lick the full span of her vaginal entrance from top to bottom, place your hand atop her mons pubis and nudge it gently toward her abdomen. This will stretch the skin and tighten her vaginal entrance, enabling you to lushly encompass her sensitive inner labia as you lick.
- As an alternative to the standard position, grab hold of her upper thighs prior to the first kiss and pivot her legs up into

the air so that only her butt is touching the bed and her vulva is completely exposed.

No matter what your approach, take it long and slow, from bottom to top, and savor every step of the journey. Now that you've lavished her with the first kiss (that long full lick), let your tongue rest flat against the length of her vaginal entrance. Encompass her vulva with your tongue. Take a moment to let the experience of the first kiss resonate.

Make sure it's *love at first lick.*

Before You Go, You Should Know

Not all kisses happen in the same context. There are frequently extenuating circumstances. To that end, take a quick glance at the Appendix if you're interested in learning more about one of the following "scenarios":

- The Protected Kiss: Learn how to put your safe-sex gear to use.
- The Scarlet Kiss: Contrary to popular opinion you can enjoy cunnilingus while she's menstruating and have a perfectly pleasurable flow-free experience.
- The Virgin Kiss: For those men and women who are brand-new to the joys of cunnilingus.
- The Pregnant Kiss: Learn how to manage the ins and outs of providing pleasure during a time when the release of sexual tension is more important than ever.

Let's Review

In this chapter we discussed the importance of the first kiss. Use it as an opportunity to express your enthusiasm about what's to come. But channel that excitement into a slow, tender kiss that lavishes the entire area of the vulva rather than just the clitoral head. Remember, when it comes to cunnilingus first impressions count.

Establishing Rhythm

A Make *and* Break Moment

YOUR FIRST KISS will leave her wanting more. It's time to show her that you can go the distance. Now is a make-or-break moment, or, as you'll soon see, a make *and* break moment—a critical juncture when many men make the mistake of sprinting for the finish line instead of pacing themselves to run a marathon.

Cunnilingus is all about the balance between movement and stillness, the counterpoint of action and reaction. *To that end, a flat still tongue pressed softly, later firmly, into her vulva will prove to be one of your most powerful positions.*

Make sure that the interval between licks is long enough to let each one resonate fully and completely. Like calling out her name in a tunnel or cave, wait until the echo has completely subsided before calling out once again. Later, as the momentum builds to a peak, action and reaction will overlap until they become virtually indistinguishable; but for now that's a ways off.

- Feel your tongue against her vulva. Let your respective nerve endings find one another and conjoin in embrace. See and feel your tongue fusing with her vulva, and then . . .
- *Break* the contact. Your tongue should completely disconnect from her vulva for a split second, causing the slightest of tremors in her pelvis: an almost imperceptible shudder of shock from the loss of your tongue. Then . . .
- *Make* contact again. As with the first kiss, take a long, slow lick from top to bottom, and lushly brush against her clitoral head with the flat broad side of your tongue.
- Then, once again, maintain a flat tongue against her vulva; don't press too hard and don't favor any one particular part. It's this "breaking and making" of contact between tongue and vulva that allows the buildup of sexual tension and will ultimately demand release through orgasm.

Build a Solid Foundation

- Get a rhythm going: long, slow lick/flat, still tongue; long, slow lick/flat still tongue. Each complete set should last about ten seconds, with five seconds on the lick and five on the flat embrace of tongue against vulva.
- Repeat this pattern for about three minutes, or fifteen to twenty complete sets.

Tongue Tip: *As you get more familiar with the routine, use your hand to push up against her mons pubis for the lick (this tightens her vaginal entrance and brings her labia closer together), and then release when you lay your tongue flat against her vulva.*

Be Alluring

- Now *avoid* the head.
- Next, vary the routine with small halfway licks, from bottom to midvagina, avoiding the area of the clitoral head altogether.
- Focus on stimulating her inner labia. This way you're not overexciting the head (remember how sensitive it is). You're teasing it, gently coaxing the head out from under its protective clitoral hood by switching your tongue strokes: from light, repetitive licks that gently graze her to deeper, halfway licks that now avoid her altogether.

Literary Lick Number One

Shakespeare wrote his plays to be performed, and there's no better audience for his poetry than her vulva. The great Bard not only inspires us, but also teaches us how to apply our tongue strokes rhythmically.

Shakespeare wrote most of his plays in verse, specifically in iambic pentameter. "Iambic" means that there is a stress on the second syllable of a word, and "pentameter" tells us that a line has five "feet," or clusters of two syllables, adding up to ten syllables in total per line.

The rhythm of iambic pentameter is simple and straightforward: da-*dum*, da-*dum*, da-*dum*, da-*dum*, da-*dum*.

Think about that rhythm as it applies to a line from Shakespeare: "Shall I/com-pare/thee to/a sum/mer's day?"

Now you're ready to let your tongue take center stage. Grab your dusty college Shakespeare off the shelf, commit a few lines to memory, and then use your tongue to iambically stimulate her clitoris. Your performance will surely garner a standing ovation.

You've alerted the clitoral head to a variation in rhythm; you've rescinded the attention that it grew accustomed to. In this way, you compel the head to find *you*, to seek out your tongue.

Smother Her in Love

Now, just when the head has been lured out from under its hood in search of the tongue that has been denied her, give it to her—smother her in it. Press the soft tip of your tongue into the head. Like a wave washing over her, bathe the head for five seconds with your wet tongue. Feel her shudder with pleasure.

> **Tongue Tip:** *As an enhancement to these routines, perform them with her legs in the air. Get a firm grip on her thighs and raise both legs so that only her butt is touching the bed. Lick her vulva tenderly and gingerly and note the tension in her legs and pelvic area as she pushes against your hands. This "pushing against a point of resistance" is a key element in developing hypertonicity—the muscular tension that contributes to sexual response and orgasmic release.*

Play the Numbers

- Go back to your halfway licks. Start with a set of five.
- Then, once again, bathe the head with the soft, wet tip of your tongue. With each complete set, increase the amount of halfway licks you apply by one, until you reach a total of ten.

This routine establishes rhythm and builds sexual tension, with just a hint of unpredictability. Most important, this routine acclimates the clitoral head to oral stimulation.

Let's Review

1. In this chapter, we discussed the importance of establishing rhythm and building a solid foundation, as well as exercising restraint when you might be tempted to apply rough passion.
2. After the first kiss, lick her vaginal entrance from top to bottom, and then rest your tongue flat against the surface of her vulva. Do this fifteen to twenty times.
3. Next lick her five times with halfway strokes, focusing on the labia and staying clear of the head. On the sixth stroke, finish the movement and press the soft tip of your tongue into her head.
4. Repeat this pattern, increasing each set of halfway licks by one until you get to ten.
5. Use this routine to establish rhythm and acclimate the head to the attentions of your tongue.

Developing Tension, Part 1

The Importance of Teamwork

NOW IT'S TIME to put some real ground behind us on the road of arousal. So far, your tongue has been leading; but now, in the spirit of good old-fashioned teamwork, let's get your fingers and hands into the action. It's all for one and one for all.

Think of your tongue, hands, and fingers as three members of a jazz trio. As with any great band, everyone has to work together in order to create beautiful music.

Deft Fingers

If, in our metaphorical trio, the tongue can be thought of as the "sax man," then your fingers are behind the piano, anchoring the tongue's rousing solos with virtuoso rhythms. Fingers collaborate with the tongue to create an array of dizzying combinations.

To begin with, let's explore the potential of a single finger and then later introduce more complex combinations. Use your index finger to:

- Flirt with her inner lips; trace the edges with your fingertip. Squeeze and pinch them playfully. Acquaint your index finger with all the diverse parts of her vulva, and take note of her responses.
- Gently stimulate her front commissure, the smooth area just above the clitoral head and hood.
- Lightly tap her frenulum, the region just below her clitoral head and above her vaginal entrance where her labia minora (inner lips) meet.
- Tease her fourchette, the area where the labia majora (outer lips) meet at the base of the vaginal entrance.
- Gently tickle the lower base of her vaginal entrance.
- As you allow your finger to wander, apply simple, steady tongue strokes. Note how the two work in combination.
- Now that you've teased her vulva, slowly insert the first two inches or so of your index finger into her vagina. Your finger should go in quite easily (assuming she's amply aroused and lubricated) and you will likely feel her interior pelvic muscles throb in response and the clitoral cuff tighten around you.
- Hold the position straight and still as you continue to apply simple tongue strokes. Don't rush to insert more fingers. Save them for later. For now, there's a teasing aspect to the still, single finger and its presence stimulates her pelvic muscles to work: you're giving her something to reach for that ultimately eludes her grasp.

A Teasing Thumb

The nublike thumb is a perfect example of the power of width over depth.

- As a playful alternative to your index finger, insert your thumb just inside her vaginal entrance, as if you're making a fingerprint. In addition to being shorter and squatter than the index finger, the thumb has more heft—so use it for shallower movements and to stimulate the surface of the vulva.

Tongue Tip: *Use your thumb in combination with your index finger. While your index finger is inserted in her vaginal entrance, rotate your thumb downward to the six o'clock position and then graze, tickle and press her perineum (the area of erectile tissue just below her vagina and above her anus). Or rotate your thumb back up to the twelve o'clock position and massage her frenulum, the area just below the clitoral head, while your finger is inserted in her vaginal entrance.*

Sturdy Hands

No jazz trio would be complete without the backup of the bass. Such is the role of your hands; not flashy like the tongue, or deft like the fingers, but nevertheless crucial in supporting the melody.

Assuming for the moment that you're right-handed, it's your left hand that will generally be employed in this supportive role, as your right hand will be focused on finger work (or vice versa if you're left-handed). Working from below, your hand provides a solid foundation for the action happening above. A firm, steady hand enables you to execute your tongue strokes with precision.

Place your free hand under her buttocks and cradle them firmly. You should be able to easily squeeze both cheeks together. Use your hand to keep her in position and fine-tune the position of her vulva in relation to your mouth. Make no mistake: a steady hand is crucial, the backbone of a great session—it helps her to easily maintain persistent contact with your mouth and allows you to modulate the pressure against her vulva.

Let's Review

1. In this chapter we commenced the process of developing sexual tension. We achieved this by introducing manual stimulation, namely in the form of a single finger inserted into the vaginal entrance. In doing so, we noted the response of her clitoral cuff and pelvic muscles.
2. We also highlighted an alternative to the index finger in the form of the thumb, as well as a playful combination in which the perineum is stimulated in combination with the index finger.
3. In addition to simple manual stimulation, we also emphasized the importance of using a hand to support her weight and keep her firmly in position. A steady grip helps you execute your tongue strokes and maintain persistent contact with her vulva.

"Time Flies"

QUESTION: "Sometimes when I'm in the middle of going down on a woman, I feel like it's never going to end. Is there any rule of thumb as to how long a cunnilingus session should last?" (Jack, 32)

ANSWER: Yes, there's a very precise answer as to how long a cunnilingus session should last—*as long as it takes to bring her to orgasm.*

That said, every woman is different when it comes to her process of sexual response, so it's difficult to accurately estimate how long a given session should last. Some women are quickly able to develop the sexual tension necessary to reach orgasm, while others require stimulation over a longer period of time.

And remember, a woman's orgasmic potential may fluctuate as a result of a wide variety of factors such as stress, exercise, diet, fatigue, medication, and alcohol (can help her to relax, but also slow her down if too much is imbibed). Broader physical factors such as age and pregnancy can also influence a woman's orgasmic potential.

It's been observed that women who masturbate regularly are often able to reach orgasm more easily during cunnilingus than those who don't. This is due to the clitoral familiarity that comes with knowing her own body and being able to navigate her way through the process of sexual response. Masturbation helps to "wire" a woman for orgasm and many women, not unlike men, are able to reach orgasm within a few minutes when pleasuring themselves (so, in theory it's possible for a man to accomplish the same with his tongue). And, of course, the degree to which a woman has been amply stimulated during foreplay also has a direct bearing on the length of a cunnilingus session.

The more confident you are in navigating her process of sexual response—the more you learn what works and what doesn't—the more efficient your experience will be.

But enough equivocating: I will offer a broad generalization and opine that *a cunnilingus session should last anywhere from fifteen to forty-five minutes on average, not including foreplay*. It's often difficult for a woman to develop the requisite sexual tension in less than fifteen minutes, and she will often become overstimulated and desensitized beyond forty-five minutes.

Brevity may be the soul of wit, but not of cunnilingus.

But rest assured: time flies when you're having fun.

Developing Tension, Part 2

Tongue Strokes

NOW THAT HER CLITORAL HEAD is fully acclimated to the attention of your tongue, it's time to vary your strokes and get playful: let your tongue take a solo. But, in doing so, remember the admonitions of Strunk and White, "Be clear. Be wild of tongue in a way we can understand!" Don't make a break with the rhythm you've established, reinforce it; play on top of it.

Horizontal Strokes

Most tongue strokes are vertical, from bottom to top, but brisk horizontal licks back and forth across the clitoral head will inflame her, particularly if they're wet and sloppy and wash over the full expanse of the head.

Diagonal Strokes

Tilt your head to the left or right (whichever is more comfortable), and press your ear against her thigh. Then lick from a lower corner point of the .clitoral region up to its diagonal opposite, brushing against the clitoral head in the process. When this is executed correctly, you'll notice that your strokes slow down because you're working harder for each one and you're using the side of your tongue as opposed to the front of it. This position may be a bit awkward on the neck, but the change in direction and pace is sure to delight her, particularly since your strokes will have a heavier, slightly sluggish quality to them. There's actually a bit of "drag" to the diagonal stroke, and within that rhythm of drag an unpredictable staccato—pleasurable tiny "spikes" that spark within her.

Tongue Tip: *Use both of your thumbs to gently part her labia minora (the smaller, inner lips) on either side and expose the clitoral head. Skim it gently with your tongue from top to bottom and left to right. Once you get the hang of it, use your index fingers to gently massage the clitoral shaft.*

Cat Licks

Ever watch a cat clean itself—repetitive and focused, consumed by the task at hand? With time to spare, a cat will clean one small patch of fur at a time, working an area over and over again before moving on. Cat licks are a staple of cunnilingus. Like a fastidious feline, work the entire vulva with short, repetitious licks. Be sure to save the clitoral head for last, and then, like a cat that's come across a trouble spot that demands a bit of extra attention, apply more focus and pressure.

Shadow Finger

Let your index finger trail behind your tongue. The hardness of your finger coming on top of your wet, soft tongue will create a pleasing contrast. Start with simple vertical and horizontal strokes, and then try more complex paths.

Flat Tongue, Still Tongue

This is one of the most underestimated and underutilized tongue positions. It's great for inducing orgasm, but more important, it's also great as a breather between tongue strokes. A flat, still tongue is like the intermission at a play, or the break between scenes. It's a chance to change the scenery and gives the actors a rest, but you're not letting the audience leave the theater. Let your tongue rest firmly and flatly against the full length of her vaginal entrance. Push your tongue into her vulva. Then let her do the work. Let her move, glide, shimmy, and grind against your tongue. Whatever she wants. Let her set the pace.

Rope-a-Dope

Think of two boxers in the ring, resting briefly in embrace during a long, grueling round. Let her pummel your resting tongue. Let her wear herself out. And then—"rope-a-dope" her! That's the strategy Muhammad Ali employed to take down George Foreman during the edge-of-your-seat "Rumble in the Jungle." Ali let Foreman clobber him for a full seven rounds. Everyone thought he was a goner. And then, when Foreman was so fatigued from pounding away that he could barely lift his tired, heavy mitts, Ali sprang to life with a lightning-fast combination that sent his dazed and confused opponent to the mat in a matter of seconds. Be like Ali. Let her push and grind against your flat, still tongue—take it all in—and then spring back with a series of fast vertical and diagonal tongue strokes. Lick

Literary Lick, Number Two

This tongue stroke pays homage to the writer Vladimir Nabokov, who wrote the classic work *Lolita* and the wonderful line, "Lo-lee-ta: the tip of the tongue taking a trip of three steps down the palate to tap, at three, on the teeth."

A lot of sex books wax enthusiastically over the virtues of writing the alphabet on a woman's vulva with one's tongue. While it sounds good on paper, it really doesn't cut it in practice.

If you're going to write the alphabet with your tongue, trace the same letter over and over, slowly and evenly.

Try writing a capital *F*, beginning with a long, solid lick from the bottom to the top, followed by a generous top sweep across the head, and culminating with a signature dash just below the clitoral hood.

Or, conversely, try a lowercase *i*, with its halfway journey up the length of her vaginal entrance and a delectable dot on the head to top it off.

Write it a hundred, if not a thousand, times, gradually increasing the force and pressure of your tongue until that letter, like an ancient hieroglyph, is indelibly inscribed in every fiber of her being.

her senseless with a short burst of energy and then return to the flat, still tongue, waiting for yet another opportune moment to spring to life again.

Suction Pucker

Pucker your lips around the clitoral glans and apply a bit of gentle suction. This technique will stimulate increased blood flow to the clitoris—an aspect of sexual response so important to female arousal that the FDA approved the Eros-CTD (Clitoral Therapy Device) for the treatment of female orgasmic disorder. This contraption consists of a small pump connected to a tiny plastic cup that fits over the head of the clitoris and is designed to simulate the effects of cunnilingus. As such, it often brings women to orgasm. Research has also suggested that the CTD pump might even prevent fibrosis of the clitoral arteries as women grow older. But there's nothing this device can do that you can't do better!

Let's Review

In this chapter we introduced some creative, playful techniques for varying the rhythm and pace of your tongue strokes. These techniques are important in that they allow you to maintain persistent clitoral contact while simultaneously mixing things up and heightening the excitement. In giving your tongue a solo, don't break the rhythm you've established, reinforce it.

Escalating the Action,
Part 1

Spot Removal

Y OU'VE UNDOUBTEDLY heard of the G-spot. You've probably spent your fair share of time searching for it, and then
wondering if you found it. But as we learned earlier, the G-spot is
much more than just a spot; in fact, to call it a spot is a serious misnomer. If anything, it's an area, a sensitive expanse. Forget the term
"G-spot" and think of it as a cluster—a clitoral cluster, that is. Think
of this cluster as the unseen "roots" of a flower that wend their way
through the "soil" of erectile tissue and pelvic bone.

Now that we know what we're looking for, let's go find it.

Come-Hither

Earlier, we explored the possibilities of manual stimulation by inserting a single, still finger into the vaginal entrance. Now incorporate slow movements of that finger into your routine:

- Start with a straight index finger and then curl it in a "come-hither" gesture.
- Gently graze her vaginal ceiling with your fingertip. As you do so, your finger will pass over the clitoral cluster, an area of sensitive spongy tissue that surrounds the urethra and swells against the vaginal ceiling when aroused. At this point in the process of arousal, her clitoral cluster should be fairly easy to find, as it is likely engorged with the inflow

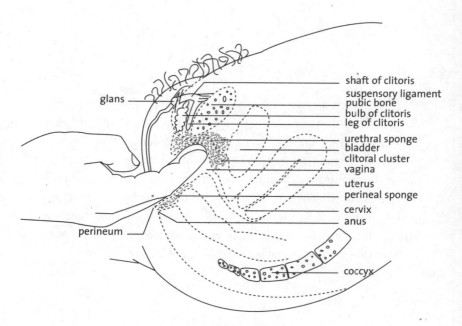

glans

perineum

shaft of clitoris
suspensory ligament
pubic bone
bulb of clitoris
leg of clitoris
urethral sponge
bladder
clitoral cluster
vagina
uterus
perineal sponge
cervix
anus

coccyx

Come-Hither Clasp

of blood. Your fingertip should end its journey in the spongy tissue where her vaginal ceiling intersects with her vaginal entrance.

- Press lightly against her pubic bone with your fingertip. She may shudder at the first touch of the area, as you are now stimulating a new hot zone in the clitoral network.
- In addition to the "come-hither" finger curl, press the length of your finger up against her vaginal ceiling—hold the position and apply pressure against the area. Don't be shy about pressing up into her vaginal ceiling. The clitoral cluster is less sensitive than the clitoral head, and responds well to firm, persistent pressure.

Tongue Tip: *As you press your finger into her vaginal ceiling, use your free hand to press down from above on her pubic mound. The pressure from above complements the pressure from below and heightens the sensitivity of the region to your touch. This is because the spongy tissue that comprises the clitoral cluster is nestled between her vaginal ceiling and pubic bone and swells against both when engorged with blood during arousal. (See the illustration at the end of this chapter for a visual of this technique.)*

- Now that you've used the come-hither finger curl to graze her vaginal ceiling/clitoral cluster, reverse position and do the same along her vaginal floor. When "trawling" her vaginal floor, you're exciting her perineal tissue (the sensitive erectile tissue that lines the expanse of skin between her vagina and anus).

Tongue Tip: *Give her a "perineal pinch." When stimulating her perineal tissue from the inside with your index finger, use your thumb to press her perineum from the outside. In this position, you're literally pinching her perineum from both sides.*

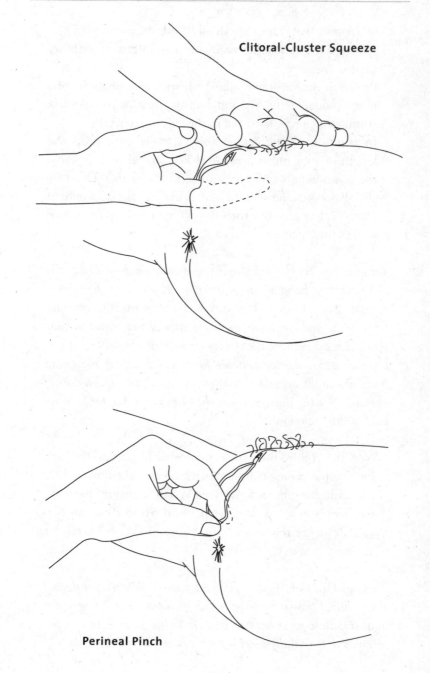

Clitoral-Cluster Squeeze

Perineal Pinch

- Having lavished attention on both the vaginal ceiling and floor, use the come-hither finger curl to graze her sensitive vaginal walls, both left and right, especially the areas that are closest to the entrance.
- Be sure to complement this manual tour of her vaginal walls with the tongue strokes described in previous chapters (vertical strokes will be the easiest and most natural). If it's too difficult to focus on performing hand *and* tongue gestures simultaneously, then simply press a flat still tongue against her clitoral head and focus on the manual stimulation.

Let's Review

In this chapter we redubbed the G-spot the clitoral cluster, expanded our definition of this important erogenous zone, and learned how to stimulate it manually with a series of finger positions.

Two's Company

NOW THAT YOU have exploited a single finger to its full potential, it's time to introduce a second finger, your middle one. Think of your index and middle fingers as a single finger and let them work in unison.

- First, simply insert both fingers inside her vaginal canal (palm up) and maintain a still position. Take a moment to feel her pelvic muscles contract against the sides of your fingers; notice the further tightening of her vaginal entrance (the clitoral cuff) around your fingers.
- As you did earlier with a single finger, use both fingers— side by side—to graze the ceiling, floor, and walls of her vagina with come-hither gestures. When grazing her vaginal ceiling, feel your fingertips pass over the spongy tissue of the clitoral cluster.

- Flatten your fingers and press them into her vaginal ceiling. Push up against the spongy tissue. Apply firm pressure. With your other hand, press down against her pubic mound.
- Use both hands to massage her from above and below.
- Continue to apply your tongue to her clitoral head—either with small vertical strokes or simply with a flat, still tongue. At this point the application of steady pressure against her clitoral head is just as important as, if not more important than, tongue strokes.
- In using both fingers and tongue, you are simultaneously engaging her clitoral cluster and clitoral head. Note that you are applying a gentle pressure to the latter and a deeper pressure to the former. The pleasure she experiences is a blend of these two types of stimulation.

The Come-Hither Clasp

- Now hook your fingertips just inside her vaginal entrance and push up against her vaginal ceiling/clitoral cluster with the tops of your fingers. Get a good firm grasp. Press your fingertips into the spongy tissue atop of her vaginal entrance, and raise the tops of your finger—through to the knuckle (or as much as comfortably possible)—against her vaginal ceiling.
- Maintain this position; apply fingertip pressure.
- Since you should still be licking her clitoral head from the outside (while stimulating it with your fingers from within), your chin should fit comfortably into the palm of your hand. Your fingertips should be pressing into the area just behind the head (only a thin layer of tissue and pelvic bone separates your fingertips and tongue).

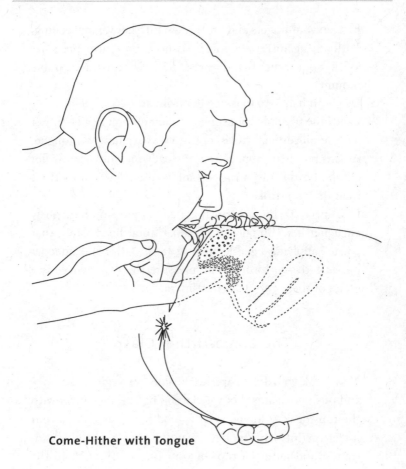

Come-Hither with Tongue

The come-hither clasp is an important position for stimulating the full expanse of her clitoral cluster as well as maintaining the position of her vulva against your mouth—it's very likely the position your fingers will be in when she reaches orgasm, with the possible addition of a third finger to round out the team and enhance the throbbing of her pelvic contractions.

Let's Review

In addition to introducing a second finger, we also illuminated the importance of the come-hither clasp—a position that enables your finger to straddle the full expanse of her clitoral cluster. At this point in the process, use your fingers to find a position and then maintain steady pressure.

An Interlude

QUESTION: "My girlfriend loves oral sex, but sometimes she complains about being lonely when I'm doing it. Is that weird?" (Rob, 29)

ANSWER: No, her sense of loneliness is not entirely uncommon. Even though cunnilingus is an intense physical experience, it's possible that she may feel a bit disconnected from you. Try straddling one of her legs so that your penis rests against her inner thigh. Stroke her stomach with your free hand. Connect more of your bodies to each other. And even though you're focused on her vulva, keep in mind that there's a whole woman up there, so make an extra effort to verbalize and stay connected.

Time-out

The come-hither clasp described in the previous chapter provides an ideal opportunity to take a quick intermission from cunnilingus and focus on other types of stimulation—assuming she'll let you.

- Still stimulating her "clitoral cluster," get up on your knees, come around to one side of her, and kiss her stomach and breasts; you can also kiss her mouth if she doesn't object, but take heed: just as the average guy doesn't always relish the idea of kissing a woman after she's gone down on him, many women would rather not kiss a wet face that has just come up from below.
- When enjoying an entr'acte, keep a small towel handy and use your free hand to give your face a quick wipe-down. You might also want to pat down her inner thighs and lightly dab her vulva.

The Perfect Pairing

A time-out also presents an opportunity to have a swish or two of wine to refresh your palate. As noted in Part I, the pH level of her vulva is remarkably similar to that of wine, so cunnilingus and the fruit of the vine are the perfect pairing. Try a dry white, or a red Zinfandel—wines that are a little more on the acidic side will add some zing to your tongue.

If you're willing to indulge your senses as well as your wallet, pick up a good bottle of Viognier from the Condrieu region in France; it possesses a rich perfume that's redolent of apricot, peaches, and honey, and, when combined with the sweet nectar of her vulva, is the closest you'll ever come to tasting ambrosia, the food of the gods. Whatever your choice, make sure you offer her a sip before go-

ing back to your tongue strokes. But remember: during this interlude, try not to remove your fingers from their come-hither clasp.
Maintain a good firm grip on her clitoral cluster and enjoy your
libations—all of them.

Let's Review

A come-hither clasp is an ideal way to take a short interlude from
cunnilingus, reconnect with her upper body, and enjoy other forms
of stimulation before returning to your session.

Escalating the Action,
Part 2

Under Pressure: The Clitoris

I T'S TIME to start applying more clitoral pressure with your mouth—*much* more. At this point in the process of sexual response, stimulation in the form of persistent pressure against the area of her clitoral head is probably the single most important element in helping her reach orgasm. The other three elements fundamental to her orgasm are:

- The rhythm of your tongue against her clitoral head
- The firm position of your fingers against her clitoral cluster
- The support of your hand under her buttocks

Taken together, these four elements enable the oral inducement of the female orgasm.

- Apply pressure with a flat, still tongue. Make your tongue as firm as possible and then press it against her clitoral head. Like a reflex, she will press her vulva into your tongue.

Now it's time to introduce a key component of oral stimulation, the "gum-press."

- Raise your upper lip by making an "Elvis Presley" snarl and press your gum against her front commissure, the sensitive area just above the head. (If you're having a problem getting the hang of exposing your gum in this manner, use your upper lip instead.)
- Start with a light pressure and adjust it accordingly to her comfort. While not as sensitive to touch as the actual clitoral head, the front commissure nevertheless abounds in nerve fibers as the clitoral shaft runs beneath it. The virtue of the gum-press is that while you apply pressure to her front commissure, you're in perfect position to easily, and skillfully, lick her head, frenulum, hood, and inner labia with your tongue.
- Similar to the flat, still tongue, let her take the lead in setting pace and rhythm. Let her use your gum as a source of resistance in order to build up the friction necessary for orgasm.

Bottom-up

When performing a gum-press, know that the pressure against your gum, at times, may prove formidable—you may even experience a slight ache—especially as she approaches orgasm.

If you feel like you need a break from the gum-press (a top-down approach), try applying pressure against her frenulum, the area just below her clitoral head. Fortunately, the frenulum, like other sensi-

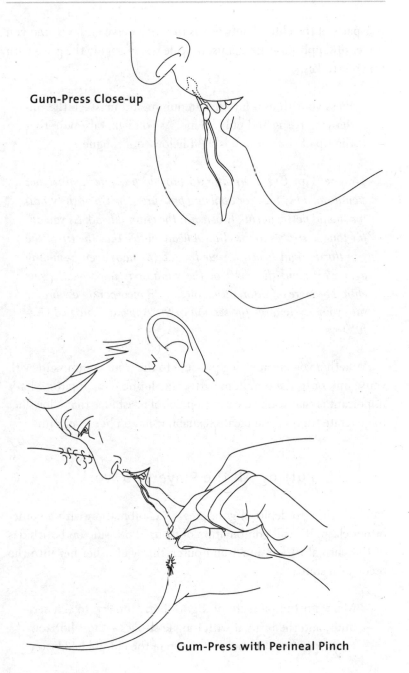

Gum-Press Close-up

Gum-Press with Perineal Pinch

tive parts of the clitoral network, is rife with nerve endings, and you can easily apply pressure against it while still engaging the glans with tongue strokes.

- Press your thumb into her frenulum and massage the underlying tissue and pubic bone. As you lick, take note that the tip of your thumb is right below your tongue.

Tongue Tip: *Use a vibrator to provide pressure against her frenulum, a key area for applying pressure. The tip of the vibrator should nestle in snugly beneath the clitoral head. As you apply tongue strokes to the clitoral head, notice that the tip of the vibrator is right beneath your tongue (perhaps even humming against it) and the shaft of the vibrator is underneath your chin. For more on information on how to incorporate a vibrator into your session, see the section in the Appendix entitled Useful Toys.*

Whether you are applying pressure to the front commissure with your gum, or to the frenulum with your thumb or a vibrator, what's important is that you're creating a point of resistance that allows her to generate friction and create sexual tension on her own terms.

Putting All the Players to Work

Now it's time to deploy a gum-press in combination with a come-hither clasp. It's this combination of focused pressure on both sides of the clitoral region, inner and outer, that will usher her into the preorgasm state.

- Maintain the pressure of a gum-press for five to ten seconds, and then vary it with tongue strokes—short horizontal passes that skim across the top of the clitoral head from left to right, or vertical strokes that hit it head-on from bottom to top.

- All the while, maintain the manual stimulation of the come-hither finger clasp.
- Get your thumb into the action by pressing it against her frenulum.
- Get your free hand (the one supporting her buttocks) into the action by stimulating her perineum. If your hand is horizontally straddling her buttocks, simply rotate it so that it's vertically aligned with the crevice between her buttocks. Now your thumb is free, willing, and able to stimulate her perineum externally.

In case you didn't know it, at this point you're working like a pro. You are stimulating the key areas of the clitoral network, both visible and hidden, and calling *all* of its parts to action!

Let's Review

1. In this chapter we discussed the importance of applying external pressure to the region around the clitoral head.
2. We introduced the technique of a gum-press against the front commissure, or alternatively fingertip or vibrator pressure against the frenulum. The point is to maintain pressure and provide a point of resistance as you continue to stimulate the clitoral head with your tongue.
3. Let her take the lead in establishing pace, rhythm, and pressure.
4. Finally, we introduced a combination that includes a come-hither clasp to stimulate the clitoral cluster; a gum-press that provides pressure against the front commissure; tongue strokes that stimulate the head; and manual stimulation of the frenulum and perineum.

A Stitch in Time

QUESTION: During a session of cunnilingus, is there anything I can do to speed up the process?

ANSWER: Whatever you do, *don't* attempt to speed things up by increasing the pace of your clitoral stimulation. One of the main complaints of women in regard to men's oral habits is that they're too fast and rough. So if you "tongue-fuck" her, or flick her clit like you're a porn star, in order to move things along, you'll likely derail the entire process and possibly even hurt her.

Also, do *not* do anything to indicate to her that you're in a rush or growing impatient. Don't sigh or groan; don't get angry or frustrated; don't glance at your watch, and certainly don't say anything like "come on, already." Refer back to the Three Assurances in Part I and take note of Assurance number two: There's no rush; she has all the time in the world. You want to savor every moment.

Remember, one of the most common anxieties women experience during cunnilingus is a fear that they're taking too long, hence the importance of this Assurance. So if she even senses that you think she might be taking too long, her anxiety may well become a self-fulfilling prophecy.

Foreplay is *the* key factor. The more a woman has been erotically stimulated during foreplay, the more easily, and quickly, she will reach orgasm. Rather than trying to decrease the time you're spending, focus on increasing the pleasure and intimacy you're providing.

Additionally, there are key moments during a session of cunnilingus when the introduction of a new element or variation—a tongue stroke, a finger, stimulation of the clitoral cluster or anus—will often hypercharge the process and take the action to the next level.

It goes without saying that a man should understand the female process of sexual response and be able to draw upon a wide variety of techniques when stimulating her. As the saying goes, "a stitch in time saves nine."

But beyond general experience, a crucial factor is often the familiarity and intuitive sense of knowing that comes from being intimately involved with a woman and learning firsthand what works and what doesn't.

Henry David Thoreau wrote, "Not that the story need be long, but it will take a long while to make it short," and the same can be said of cunnilingus. In order to create a short work—one that has all the power and resonance of a longer one—you must know your craft as well as your subject. And such intimate knowledge comes with time, practice, and dedication.

Preorgasm, Part 1

ONCE HER ORGASM was but a distant and faraway destination in your journey down the road of arousal. Now the contours of her skyline are plainly in view, the throbbing pulse of Main Street tangible. You've just entered the city limits. Welcome to Orgasmopolis!

The Visible Signs of Arousal

When it comes to sex and the "moment after," perhaps the single most frequently asked question by men is, "Uh . . . did you come?" To many guys, the female orgasm is a mystery, a conundrum: a chimera so intangible and elusive that they often fail to recognize it when it's happening right before their very eyes.

Shortly, we will examine *precisely* what occurs when a woman is experiencing an orgasm. But for now, rest assured—if you are in tune with her process of sexual response, if you're in lockstep all the way, then you will notice visible signs of the impending climax well before the event itself. These indications will be most apparent in the preorgasm phase, the moments just preceding her orgasmic contractions.

So what are the visible signs of arousal? How can you tell when she's close to orgasm?

Throughout the ages wise men have reflected upon this question and, in *The Tao of Love and Sex*, author Jolan Chang offers us the "indications of female arousal" as laid out by Taoist master Wu Hsien:

1. She is panting and her voice is shaking uncontrollably.
2. She closes her eyes and her nostrils are widened and she is unable to speak.
3. She is staring at the man.
4. Her ears turn red and her face is flushing, but the tip of her tongue turns slightly colder.
5. Her hands are hot and her abdomen warm, and at the same time her language becomes almost unintelligible.
6. Her expression looks as though she is bewitched, her body is soft as jelly, and her limbs are droopy.
7. The saliva under her tongue has been sucked dry and her body is pressing against the man.
8. The pulses of her vulva become noticeable and her secretions are flowing.

Well, okay. While today's modern man might not notice that "the saliva under her tongue has been sucked dry," he is—as evidenced by the medley of quotes below—apt to observe:

"I feel her vagina tighten. It starts to throb and pulse, like the beating of her heart."

"Her body stiffens, her muscles tighten. She flexes and releases, flexes and releases—especially her legs."

"Her skin flushes; her entire body heats up."

"She starts perspiring."

"Her abdominal muscles tighten."

"Her breasts swell."

"I notice a difference in her taste; her juices start to thicken, they get sweeter and warmer. It's like they're being heated up from all the action, roiling in a cauldron."

"She holds me tightly in position and won't let me move."

"She locks me in."

"Her breathing gets really deep, like she's running a marathon."

"I feel her heart racing, pounding."

"She starts grabbing at my hair and ears."

"She pushes up her pelvis."

"She grinds against me."

"She bites her lower lip."

"She tells me, 'Keep going, keep going; don't stop.'"

"She finds something to grab—my hair, a finger, a piece of blanket."

"She enters another world. She's completely lost in concentration."

"It's like she's possessed and speaking in tongues."

Ninety Seconds Away

Cunnilinguists are in a great position to observe the visible signs of arousal, especially when the lights are on. Of particular note will be the darkening in color and deepening in luster of her inner labia, as well as the retraction of the clitoral head into its hood—*both are signs that she's within ninety seconds of reaching climax.* Even in the dark, it's not hard to observe when the glans has retracted; focus on feeling the head when it's fully protruded and erect, and you'll easily be able to recognize its absence.

Let's Review

In this chapter, we discussed the visible signs of arousal, and how to determine when she's within ninety seconds of orgasm.

Preorgasm, Part 2

Stay in Position

ONE of the most challenging aspects of the preorgasm phase is simply holding her in place and helping her to maintain the position of her clitoris against your mouth. What's ahead of her is a straightaway, and you need to make sure that she stays on track and there are no sudden turns. Too often a woman loses hold of an orgasm just before it's about to happen. You need to be consistent as well as persistent.

Think about it: a very small area (the region of her clitoral head) needs to maintain persistent, forceful contact with another very small area (your tongue and gum). Without your hands holding her tightly in position (one under her butt, the other inside her vaginal entrance), without your mouth and gum pressed into her clitoral area and without the methodic, rhythmic sweeps of your tongue, her orgasm will fast lose its inevitability and become a mere possibility. Think of yourself as helping to keep her clitoris positioned between a rock and a hard place.

- Once she's in the preorgasm phase, bring her legs close together. In this position it's much easier for her pelvic muscles to transition into an involuntary state of spasm. If her legs are too wide apart, she may not be able to orgasm at all. Don't worry about not having enough space to stimulate her with your tongue—there's plenty of room. Remember, her clitoral head is an *external* part of her vulva and closer to the surface of the mons pubis than the inside of the vagina.
- In this position, everything narrows and tightens—the walls of her vagina around your fingers, her legs around your arms—all activity becomes constrained and more concentrated. To an outside observer, it may look as though you're both rather still, but, in fact, all you need do is loosen your grip ever so lightly to unleash a veritable whirlwind of movement.

Let's Review

In this chapter, we discussed the importance of helping her maintain position. Focus on keeping her as still as possible and constraining her movements. Also, make sure her legs are as close together as possible.

Posterior Pizzazz

CONSIDER SPICING UP the action with a bit of anal play. Remember: the clitoris and anus are connected through perineal tissue and the sphincter contracts during orgasm along with the pelvic muscles. In short, the anal region participates in the process of sexual response and is connected to the clitoral network.

As with all elements of cunnilingus, a little goes a long way, and anal stimulation is no exception. Like everything else we've discussed, it's about stimulation rather than penetration.

- Thus far, you've stimulated the perineum and the area just around her anus. Now graze the anus with your fingertip and then insert it—just the fingertip. As soon as you penetrate her anal area, you should feel the tightening of her sphincter muscles against your finger.
- Hold this position through her orgasm.

Tongue Tip: *When stimulating the anus, you may need some of that lubricant you've been keeping on hand. Typically, it won't be necessary, as some of the moisture from her vulva has naturally made its way south to the perineum and into the anal area, but it doesn't hurt to be prepared.*

- When stimulating the anus, make sure to insert a finger that's not employed in manual stimulation of the vulva, as there are bacteria in the former that you don't want coming into contact with the latter. Your best bet is the thumb of your hand that's supporting her buttocks. You should be able to position yourself easily so that you're able to support her buttocks in addition to inserting the *tip* of your thumb into her anus.
- Or insert the pinkie or fourth finger of the hand that is involved in manual stimulation—those two fingers are usually neglected anyway during manual stimulation of the vulva, so give them some active duty.

It's worth noting that while cunnilingus is a generally accepted form of sexual expression, stimulating the anal area is sometimes considered off-limits, even though there's a big difference between a wee fingertip in the butt and full-blown anal intercourse. If it's your first time, tease the general environs a bit with your finger and be sure to give her clear physical cues that you're "approaching and entering." If she's uncomfortable, then pull back; it's not worth jeopardizing a productive cunnilingus session over.

Let's Review

In this chapter we discussed the role that the anal area plays in the process of sexual response and the type of stimulation that's best deployed in conjunction with cunnilingus. Once again, think about stimulation as opposed to penetration. Anal stimulation can seriously enhance the quality of her orgasm, but if overdone, it can also detract.

Preorgasm, Part 3

A S SHE TEETERS close to orgasm, take a moment to get into a cool, calm headspace. Don't get swept away by all the excitement. One of the main advantages of cunnilingus over intercourse is that you can remain levelheaded and in control throughout the entire experience; the most common mistake men make is to meet passion with passion. Having come this far, do NOT let the cunnilingus session degenerate into random chaos in the penultimate moments.

Cool, Calm Tongue Strokes

Now is the ideal time to *play it cool* with your tongue, maybe even a little hard to get. The smaller and lighter your tongue strokes, the more you will prolong the heightened sensations just prior to orgasm and build sexual tension.

- If you're licking her with rhythmic, vertical strokes, try skipping one. For example: 1-2-3-4, 1-2-skip-4; or 1-skip-2-skip, 1-skip-2-skip.
- Or introduce a horizontal swipe amid a series of vertical strokes—just as we began the cunnilingus session with some teasing, so too can we end it that way.
- Slow down. Let her orgasm come to you. Tease it out of her. Not only will this teasing help to trigger her orgasm, it will also sharpen the orgasmic contractions.

Here are three creative techniques to calmly coax her orgasm:

Jackson Pollock Licks

A bit of lore about the painter Jackson Pollock: a journalist came to his studio one afternoon, surveyed the artist's work and, unimpressed by the abstract splotches, told him, "That's not art, any monkey can do that." Pollock dipped his brush in a can of paint, gave it a deft flick of the wrist, and told the journalist to get the hell out. He pointed to the doorknob: on it, dead center, was a single dot of paint.

- Try licking her the way Pollock painted: broad strokes, with pinpoint targeted precision. Swooping, serpent like, start with the flat part of the tongue and end with the tip. Like Pollock, be sure you know what you're aiming for; demonstrate the precision that underlies the passion.

The Lily Pad

Imagine a frog on a lily pad. It sits silently and patiently, and then suddenly its tongue darts out to snag its prey. Make like a frog and "catch" the clitoral head with your tongue. In cunnilingus, less is definitely more, and this technique—with its pauses and sudden flashes of contact—bears that out.

Finishing Touches

Impressionist painter Georges Seurat pioneered the art of "pointil-lism"—rendering his subject out of thousands, if not millions, of tiny dots of color. Like Seurat proudly surveying a barely dry land-scape, apply a few considered finishing touches to your "canvas"—using the tiniest tongue tip of a brush, liven up your subject with a burst of pointed color.

G et ready: here comes the first of a series of involuntary, spas-modic contractions that signal she's reached orgasm and is about to release the tension that you both worked so hard to build.

As Masters and Johnson noted of the preorgasm phase, or what they called the plateau phase, "The female gathers psychological and physiological strength from the stockpile of mounting sexual tension, until she can direct all her physical and mental forces to-ward a leap into the third, or orgasmic phase, of sexual tension ex-pression."

Let's Review

In this chapter, we discussed the value of small, light tongue strokes as she approaches orgasm. These tiny gestures provide contrast to the pressure of your gum against her front commissure; they also help to prolong the last heightened phase of preorgasm and build further sexual tension.

A Note for Those Stuck
Without an Ending

SOMETIMES a woman is simply unable to reach orgasm via cunnilingus and will founder in the preorgasm phase unless there's a transition into genital intercourse. This may occur for a variety of reasons:

- She may be under the impression that intercourse is the proper, or only, way in which a woman should experience orgasm.
- She may be uncomfortable with the idea of coming in a man's mouth.
- Or perhaps she simply hasn't "trained" her body to experience an orgasm in this manner.

As Natalie Angier wrote, "The intimate connection between a woman's psychic humor and her clitoral power means that the clitoris must be wired up to the brain—the big brain—before it can sing. The brain must learn to ride its little rod the way it must learn to balance its body on a bicycle. And once learned, the skill will not be forgotten."

Most women have "wired" themselves to orgasm consistently through masturbation and then subsequently settle for the inconsistency of genital intercourse. Since many men do not, as a rule, use their tongues to take a woman through the *entire* process of sexual response, many women are not "wired" to come as a result of cunnilingus.

Fortunately, such modification is easily achieved. Reassure her, let her relax into the process; let her know that you want her to come in this manner; let her know how much you're enjoying it. Give her time to feel her way through the process, and don't fret if she doesn't come the first time. She'll get there as long as you're providing the stimulation she needs.

But if she still insists on genital intercourse, make sure the transition to penetration is seamless. It's all too easy to lose the rhythm that's been established and squander all that sexual tension you've so carefully gathered.

For more on this subject, refer to Chapter Forty-three.

The Female Orgasm: Expanding Your Vocabulary

LET'S POLISH UP on our vocabulary, and meanwhile learn a thing or two about the female orgasm:

WORD: *"Rabelaisian"*

DEFINITION: like Rabelais or his writings; marked by exuberant imagination and caricature.

EXAMPLE: "The walls trembled violently from the shouts of her orgasm—so much so that the man wondered if her ululations weren't more *Rabelaisian* than real."

In 1994, Shere Hite observed that more than half the women in her latest survey were faking orgasm, with only 42 percent getting there with a male partner. More recently, some studies have put the number of women who don't orgasm consistently as high as 58 percent. *The best way to know if a woman's faking an orgasm is by knowing how to recognize the real thing.*

To an informed cunnilinguist, in tune with her process of sexual response, this is easier than you might suspect. As we discussed earlier, there are visible signs of arousal that become apparent throughout the process of sexual response, particularly during the preorgasm phase.

These include:

- An increase in the pace of her breathing
- An increase in body temperature and heart rate
- A high state of tension in her muscles, also known as hypertonicity
- A tightening of the abdominal muscles
- The throbbing of her PC muscles, and a general "bearing down" on the pelvic area

In addition to observing these visible signs of arousal during the preorgasm phase, *you will principally recognize the female orgasm through the spasmodic, involuntary contractions of her genital area, also known as pelvic thrusting.*

- As she releases sexual tension through orgasm, her vagina and uterus will contract, on average, ten to fifteen times, with each contraction lasting approximately eight tenths of a second; her rectal sphincter contracts anywhere from two to five times as well. Based on these measurements, the average female orgasm lasts anywhere from ten to twenty seconds.
- Attendant to these genital and rectal contractions is the tensing and releasing, in spasm, of many of the muscles throughout her body, including arms, legs, neck, and face—even her toes will bend and arch forward.

- During orgasm, her breathing will speed up and her pulse will soar (anywhere from 110 to 180 beats per minute).
- In some cases, a woman may ejaculate a clear fluid.

Tongue Tip: *If you're wondering if her orgasm was the real McCoy, look for the increased prominence of her nipples. It may appear that they are becoming more erect, but in actuality the area of her areolas is subsiding to its normal state. Another sign of her orgasm is the rapid subsiding of her "sex flush" and the appearance of a filmy sheen of perspiration in its place.*

One way of thinking about the female orgasm is not as an action, but rather as a *reaction*, the involuntary release of all the sexual tension she built up throughout the process of arousal and the final surrender and letting go. It's important to remember that no two women are the same when it comes to their orgasms, and many sex therapists consider the individual experience so unique that it's sometimes referred to as "orgasmic fingerprinting."

That said, there are consistencies in the overall structure of an orgasm, with the average woman experiencing a sudden sense of "stopping," followed immediately by intense, sharp contractions, which gradually slow and wane into a duller, more blunted, pelvic throbbing before subsiding.

Back to the question of how to tell when she's faking it. Many women can duplicate the characteristics of orgasm, including the contractions of the PC muscles, although it's unlikely she could manufacture eight to ten of these contractions in less than twenty seconds, especially in combination with all the other visible characteristics. In fact, some sex therapists will recommend to women who have trouble experiencing orgasms that they do just that—fake their way through one in order to stimulate and trick the body into experiencing the real thing.

But, in truth, most women know that they needn't bother portraying a convincing facsimile of the real thing when they can simply offer up an ersatz performance of those characteristics that are most likely to fool and please *men*. In short, lots of sound and fury, which, in the end, is nothing more than smoke and mirrors. This is a broad generalization, but it's the *screamers* and the *thrashers* who are very often the *fakers*.

An orgasm doesn't come out of nowhere; it's the final exclamation point on a sentence that you've been writing all along. If the final flourish feels unearned, then it likely is.

WORD: *"Coadjutor"*

DEFINITION: a helper, assistant.

EXAMPLE: "As a loyal and diligent *coadjutor* in the satisfaction of his mistress, he knew exactly what to do as her body began to spasm and shudder with pleasure."

When a woman enters the period of orgasmic contractions, stay absolutely focused on what you're doing. Maintain your position. Provide a steady point of resistance. Feel the contractions of her orgasm, the thrusting of her pelvis. Like a shock absorber, take her movements into your body and then channel them back into her in the form of pleasurable vibrations. Contain the energy; smother it. Let it out slowly. Don't let the orgasm explode out of her in one quick, furious blast; tease it out slowly in long, fluid pulses.

Stay calm and cool. Now's not the moment to get caught up in

Wait until she's come to a complete stop! Whereas men reach a point of "ejaculatory inevitability" during the process of sexual response, also known as the point of no return, women require persistent, unbroken clitoral stimulation even as they are in the midst of climaxing, lest the orgasm come to a grinding halt.

the hullabaloo and lose your discipline. Soon enough it will be your turn. *Make sure you finish what you've started.*

It's all too easy to confuse the moments just prior to her orgasm with the orgasm itself. The female orgasm is preceded by small, growing waves of pleasure that ebb and build, and these waves may have the appearance of an orgasm. She's in the process of coming, without having actually peaked yet. Her pelvic area is throbbing, but she hasn't yet gone into the involuntary state of spasmodic release. When the actual orgasm happens, it will break the rhythm that precedes it; there's a brief violence to the moment—a spasm, a shudder—like that first jolt when the wheels of a landing plane touch the runway. The actual orgasm may only last ten to twenty seconds at its peak; but the entire process—replete with spine-tingling ebbs and flows—may easily last several minutes.

WORD: *"Appoggiatura"*

MEANING: an embellishment: a musical note performed before an essential part of a melody and normally taking half or less than half its time value.

EXAMPLE: "When a woman climaxes as a result of oral stimulation, one can deftly apply small, yet highly effective *appoggiaturas* that enhance and punctuate the larger experience."

If, and when, a woman climaxes during genital intercourse, you may feel the contractions of her orgasm pulse against your penis, but there's little you can do to stimulate or enhance those pleasurable waves beyond maintaining persistent contact with her clitoris.

However, during cunnilingus, you have the added benefit of being able to use your tongue to "spike" the process.

- Once she's entered the period of orgasmic contractions—about ten to twenty seconds in duration—apply light, playful tongue jabs against the clitoral head; swipe the head with short vertical strokes, mixed in with some diagonal swipes. As always, do this calmly, coolly, and gently. These "appoggiaturas" should be light tongue tickles that go against the grain of her orgasm. Think of them as tiny bumps in the road: they won't slow her down, but she'll definitely feel them. Take your time: you needn't apply more than four to six swipes in total. Each one will add spark and counterpoint to the process—power spikes that continue to push the envelope of pleasure until all the sexual tension has been completely exhausted and drained from her body. In short, use your tongue to tease out every last bit of pleasure.

WORD: *"Anfractuous"*
MEANING: full of twists and turns.
EXAMPLE: "So *anfractuous* was the process of arousing her, so dizzying and roundabout his journey, that even after the last of her fitful contractions subsided, he still wasn't sure she was fully sated."

You'll know her climax has concluded when her body relaxes, her breathing slows, and the contractions, like an echo, have faded into the distance. It will seem as though she's melted blissfully right before your eyes. Her genitals, particularly the clitoral head, will be so sensitive from the experience that she'll recoil at their slightest touch. Stimulate her until she reaches the point where she can no longer bear the touch of your tongue. She may signal this moment by placing a hand on your head, or gently pushing you away. Take the cue, and lift your head.

It's a job well done. But by no means over.

Moreplay: She Comes Again (and Again)

"It's pure instinct. The curtain comes down
when the rhythm seems right—when
the action calls for a finish."
—Harold Pinter

"Great is the art of the beginning,
but greater is the art of the ending."
—Thomas Fuller

YOU'LL FIND THAT one of the great joys of adopting the philosophy of *She Comes First* is not only that she experiences orgasm *consistently* during sexual activity, but also, when you postpone your orgasm until after hers, that the door is now open for her to experience many, many more.

In fact, it's *far easier* for a woman to experience her second orgasm, as her genitals are still engorged with blood and her body is still awash with the potent chemicals of sex. As Natalie Angier has written of the female orgasm, "It may take many minutes to reach the first summit, but once there the lusty mountaineer finds wings awaiting her. She does not need to scramble back to the ground before scaling the next peak, but can glide like a raptor on currents of joy."

Easier said than done. As far as the average guy is concerned, if stimulating a *single* female orgasm is already something of a mys-

The authors of *Sex: A Man's Guide* cite a study conducted at the University of Wisconsin in which it was found that women who were multiorgasmic were more likely to have partners who delayed their orgasms until after the women had their first ones.

tery, the whole idea of *multiple* orgasms is like the riddle of the Sphinx. More often than not men tend to think that a woman's potential to experience multiple orgasms has something to do with a "special capacity" or "unique ability" within *her*, and little or nothing to do with him: either she can or she can't.

Well, the truth is that most women *can* experience multiple orgasms—as a rule not an exception—and it has *everything* to do with you. But rest assured: if you can get her to her first orgasm, you should be able to get her to her second. Most women don't experience their second or third orgasm with men for the same reason that many don't experience their first—they're not receiving appropriate clitoral stimulation and male gratification is not being postponed.

But just because she's not having multiple orgasms with you doesn't mean she's not having them at all. Most women are able to achieve multiple orgasms during masturbation. In fact, Masters and Johnson found that some women were able to reach fifty consecutive orgasms with a vibrator! It's not that women are doing anything "special" in order to achieve multiple orgasms when masturbating, they're simply providing themselves with the focused clitoral stimulation they require.

The innate biological capacity to achieve multiple orgasms has much to do with how women, following to orgasm, experience the resolution period and return to the prearoused state. Men lose their erections quickly and go into what's called a refractory period (an interval of time that needs to pass before he can get an erection again), but a woman's genitals take far longer to return to their normal state, at least five to ten minutes. Additionally, the clitoris does not contain a venous plexus, the mechanism in the penis for retaining blood and sustaining an erection—a critical element in the explosive male orgasm and the process of insemination.

If you want to lead a woman to her second orgasm and beyond, first return to the activities of foreplay—kissing, embracing, and soft touching. Keep her warm, keep her aroused, but take some time before returning to more intense genital stimulation. (Remember, unlike other parts of her body, the clitoris—particularly the head—is extremely sensitive after orgasm.) Give yourself some time to cool down as well and recover from the excitement of what has just passed. Once you're both ready for genital stimulation, you can do so with your hands, tongue, or even your penis. That's right: there's a time and a place for everything, and the time for intercourse is *after* she's experienced her first orgasm—not simply because she's been satisfied once, but because in this "warmer" state of arousal, she's much more likely to experience a second one.

Seamless Transitions

BEFORE TRANSITIONING to genital penetration, use cunnilingus as a way of bringing her as near as possible to the point of orgasmic inevitability.

Woman on Top

Once she's there, try the *female superior* position, or woman on top. This is an ideal position for her to:

- Position her clitoris against your pubic bone at the base of your penis and achieve the ideal amount of pressure
- Stimulate her clitoral cluster against your penis
- Control rhythm and pace
- Modulate the experience of orgasm

According to Masters and Johnson, "Clitoral response may develop more rapidly and with greater intensity in the female-superior coition than in any other female coital positions." Additionally, when she's on top, you're doing less thrusting and are, therefore, more likely to be able to control the timing of your own orgasm.

The Coital Alignment Technique (CAT)

This is a sexual position designed to greatly improve a woman's chance of orgasm through genital penetration and function as an enhancement to the standard missionary position, man on top. During CAT, the man penetrates from a higher angle than usual, placing pressure on the woman's clitoris with the base of his penis and pubic bone. When you are performing CAT, the main thing to keep in mind is maintaining contact with the clitoris. The overall movement is much less a thrusting than a synchronized rocking back and forth with the focus on the clitoris and the base of the penis.

Achieving Simultaneity

PERHAPS YOU'VE MADE the decision to pursue a simultaneous orgasm. If you need to build up momentum during her "orgasmic peak" in order to achieve your own, do so through a "rocking" motion that keeps the base of your penis and pubic bone aligned with her clitoris.

Don't feel pressure to be overly inventive. The ability to achieve simultaneity often comes from the intuitive sense of knowing and understanding that develops in a committed relationship. From this perspective, it should come as no surprise that, according to the *Sex in America* survey, three out of four of married women say they always or usually reach climax during sex, compared to fewer than two out of three of single women. In large part, the success of the married vs. the unmarried comes from an understanding of each other's body and the knowledge of what works and what doesn't.

In this sense, in a committed relationship one experiences the joy of repetition. You are no longer focused on learning how to satisfy; you know how to satisfy. You don't need to think about it. In this loss of self-consciousness, you can trust your bodies to find their way to mutual pleasure, and, in doing so, release yourselves to a purer state of sexual being.

Kierkegaard wrote, "Hope is a charming maiden that slips through the fingers, Recollection is a beautiful old woman but of no use at the instant, Repetition is a beloved wife of whom one never tires."

Whether married or not, great sex often comes from the appreciation of repetition and the enjoyment of what you have.

Don't Forget Your Epilogue

ALMOST EVERY GREAT WORK of dramatic art follows its climax with a return to order, a restoration of balance, and a sense of closure. Sometimes it's just a short scene, a single instant, a brief ride off into the sunset, but in that flash of a moment we are left with a pervasive sense of calm and well-being, a comforting feeling that all is right with the world. In this sense, the experience is never really over.

A great session of sex, oral or genital, is no different. After the hurly-burly and hullabaloo of the climax—the denouement of our respective orgasms—we need to establish a moment of calm, a period of rest, a settling of the ground beneath us. To put it bluntly: when all is said and done, don't just roll over or get up and head to the fridge. Just because you've both experienced your fill of orgasms doesn't mean the play process is over. Just as you put fifteen minutes or more into foreplay, you need to put some quality time into moreplay. Don't get caught in the snuggle gap! Whether you hold each other in embrace, kiss and touch, or simply talk, moreplay is about staying connected. Moreplay is not rolling over and going to sleep, or jumping out of bed to make that "important" phone call.

To borrow a phrase from the pioneering sexologist Theodore Van de Velde, it's in the moments subsequent to orgasm when a man proves whether or not he's an "erotically civilized" adult.

Don't put a damper on an otherwise brilliant performance. An extra fifteen minutes spent cuddling, snuggling, and whispering sweet nothings is the path to greatness, the road to the sexual "big leagues"; whereas coming and then *going* is a one-way ticket to Palookaville.

Don't take this moment for granted. Stay focused, and stay connected. Ride off into the sunset together. And get ready for a brave new dawn . . .

PART

Putting It All Together

THREE

The Substance of Style

A S YOU VENTURE FORTH into an *amazing* session of cunnilingus—thoroughly acquainted with her sexual anatomy; equipped with an understanding of her process of response; and versed in a range of techniques for stimulating her—remember:

- Make sure she's amply aroused. Spend the time during foreplay to establish a strong foundation of sexual tension.
- Before you apply the first oral kiss, make sure you're both in positions that can be sustained comfortably throughout the entire process of sexual response.
- When applying your oral techniques, focus on stimulation rather than penetration. Apply gentle, rhythmic tongue strokes. Remember: all those sensitive nerve endings that contribute to her orgasm are right there at the tip of your tongue.

- Express the Three Assurances of cunnilingus persistently throughout your session: 1) Going down on her turns *you* on; you enjoy it as much as she does. 2) There's no rush; she has all the time in the world; you want to savor every moment. 3) Her scent is provocative, her taste intoxicating: it all emanates from the same beautiful essence.
- When using your fingers, don't probe and prod; focus on fingertip pressure of key areas such the clitoral cluster.
- Remember the virtues of the flat, still tongue. Stillness can be more effective than movement.
- Be confident, not cocky. A simple, modest approach is much more effective than a flashy one.
- Cunnilingus is not something you do *to* her; it's something you do with her. Let her move against you to create the friction she needs.
- As she approaches orgasm, maintain persistent clitoral contact. Keep her legs as close together as possible while still permitting access to her vulva.
- Stay calm, measured, and focused. Don't lose the process; don't let her orgasm get away from you.
- As she's coming, embellish and extend the contractions of her orgasm with light tongue strokes.
- Always finish what you started. Cunnilingus is a complete process with a beginning, middle, and end.
- The experience isn't over just because she's had an orgasm. Whether you lead her to one orgasm or to many, return together to the prearoused state.

Most important, your style begins and ends with *who* you are, rather than with what you do or how you do it. Just as no two women will respond in the same way to the techniques described in this book, no two men will apply them in quite the same way.

Routines: A Cheat Sheet

ERE YOU WILL FIND a series of routines (from beginner to advanced) that integrate and unify many of the techniques described in each phase of coreplay. These routines were not designed to be committed to memory, but rather to demonstrate how the techniques can be put into action to create a seamless session of cunnilingus. In the appendices is a blank template that you can Xerox and use to create your own routines.

When pulling it all together and implementing specific techniques, keep in mind the key elements you've learned that will guide your overall approach to composition. These elements of composition include:

- The stimulation of ten key hot spots: clitoral head and hood; mons pubis; clitoral cluster; front commissure and

clitoral shaft; frenulum; labia minora; vaginal entrance; the fourchette perineum; the anus
- Over the course of six key stages: the first kiss; establishing rhythm; developing tension; escalation; preorgasm; orgasm
- Using three main "actors": tongue; fingers; hands
- And a variety of "supporting actors": gums; penis (optional); sex toys and restraints (also optional; see appendices)

If you are a newcomer to cunnilingus, see the Q&A section entitled the Virgin Kiss in the Appendix. Also, in building your initial routines focus on simple tongue strokes, and experiment with using your tongue and fingers in combination. Most important, take a *pleasure-oriented* approach, not an *orgasm-focused* one, and observe what works and what doesn't.

If you're in the "intermediate" phase, focus on getting your tongue and hands working together and stimulating all aspects of the clitoral network, including internal areas such as the clitoral cluster. Additionally, stay attuned to her process of response and embellish her orgasm. Develop the proficiency to lead her consistently to orgasm, and make sure it's the result of comprehensive clitoral stimulation.

If you're in the "advanced" phase, experiment with unique new approaches that push the envelope in terms of fusing technique and intuition. Additionally, lead her down the path of multiple orgasms and integrate a simultaneous one into your crescendo.

When building your routines, let the key elements of composition guide your choices—in this way, the techniques you employ are sure to add up to a whole that is greater than the sum of its parts.

Routines: Beginner to Advanced

ROUTINE 1

This is a basic beginner's routine that will familiarize the newcomer with fundamental tongue strokes. It will keep finger work to bare minimum and encourage the observation of sexual response.

► *Level: Beginner* ◄

► **Stage 1: First Kiss**
(less than one minute)

TONGUE: Long, slow tongue stroke; bottom to top. Be as light and gentle as possible.

HAND: Both hands under buttocks, legs partially separated. Firm grip.

▶ Stage 2: Establishing Rhythm
(three to five minutes)

TONGUE: Vertical halfway licks (5), followed by long tongue stroke that brushes clitoral head. Focus on labia and frenulum; only brush clitoral head on full stroke, not halfway ones.

FINGERS: Single finger (index) inserted partially into vaginal entrance.

HAND: Move one hand out from under butt in order to insert finger. Use one hand to get a firm grip and straddle both cheeks.

▶ Stage 3: Developing Tension
(five to ten minutes)

TONGUE: Alternate vertical strokes of the tongue with horizontal strokes. On vertical strokes, try to just graze bottom of the clitoral head without fully hitting it. Focus on brushing the head on horizontal strokes. For every five vertical, do one horizontal.

FINGERS: Maintain single finger in vaginal entrance. Focus on feeling pelvic muscles. Let your other fingers graze vulva and perineum.

HAND: Maintain support.

Stage 4: Escalation
(three to five minutes)

TONGUE: Continue vertical and horizontal strokes. Integrate tongue press against clitoral head. Hold for five seconds.

FINGERS: Insert second finger into vaginal entrance. Press fingers against vaginal ceiling. Feel for clitoral cluster.

HAND: As you support buttocks, straddling both cheeks, try to stimulate perineum with your thumb.

Stage 5: Preorgasm
(three to five minutes)

TONGUE: Press tongue into clitoral head. Focus on pressure, slow down tongue stroke as you provide resistance. Let her move against your tongue.

FINGERS: With two fingers inserted (palm up), use your thumb to press against frenulum and provide requisite pressure. Keep fingers inside, but make sure that thumb against frenulum is your priority.

HAND: Use your hand to support buttocks and maintain clitoral contact; keep her in position. Make sure her legs are close together. You should feel her inner thighs press against your hand that is inserted in vaginal entrance.

Stage 6: Orgasm
(less than one minute)

TONGUE: Focus on pressing your tongue into clitoral head. Feel her push against you. Maintain pressure. Observe orgasmic contractions and hold in position throughout. After contractions, lick clitoral head once lightly. She should recoil to touch.

FINGERS Feel pelvic muscles throb against fingers. Focus on maintaining pressure with thumb against frenulum.

HAND: Focus on maintaining position as she enters period of spasmodic orgasmic contractions. Use your hand to press up against buttocks and keep clitoral head aligned with tongue.

COMMENTS: Focus on observing the process of sexual response and learning how your tongue stimulates reaction. Remember to be gentle and slow with your tongue and don't overstimulate the clitoral head too early in the process. Toward the end, remember to let her establish rhythm and move against you and to focus on keeping her in position as you maintain direct clitoral contact through final orgasm. If need be, incorporate a vibrator into routine in lieu of fingers, and focus on tongue strokes.

ROUTINE 2

This routine will largely maintain the tongue strokes of the last routine, but also focus on integrating fingers and gums more fully.

▶ *Level: Beginner* ◀

Stage 1: First Kiss
(less than one minute)

TONGUE: Long, slow tongue stroke; bottom to top. Be as light and gentle as possible.

FINGERS: With the hand you will use for finger work, press down on pubic mound and tighten vaginal entrance.

HAND: Other hand under buttocks; press thumb against perineum.

Stage 2: Establishing Rhythm
(three to five minutes)

TONGUE: Vertical halfway licks (5), followed by long tongue stroke that brushes clitoral head. Focus on labia and frenulum; only brush clitoral head on full stroke, not halfway ones.

FINGERS: Maintain pressure on pubic mound, keeping vaginal entrance tight and clitoral head more exposed to tongue strokes.

HAND: With one hand under buttocks, continue to use your thumb to press against perineum.

Stage 3: Developing Tension
(five to ten minutes)

TONGUE: Alternate vertical strokes with horizontal strokes. On vertical strokes, try to just graze bottom of clitoral head without fully hitting it. Focus on brushing head on horizontal strokes. For every five vertical, do one horizontal.

FINGERS: Single finger (index) inserted partially into vaginal entrance; as you apply tongue strokes, focus on moving your index finger in come-hither motion against vaginal floor, ceiling, and left and right wall. Also focus on clasping clitoral cluster on vaginal ceiling for longer intervals as well as perineal tissue at vaginal floor.

HAND: Maintain support and thumb press against perineum.

Stage 4: Escalation

(three to five minutes)

TONGUE: Press gum or upper lip into front commissure. Continue vertical and horizontal strokes.

FINGER: Insert second finger into vaginal entrance, and continue to rotate come-hither strokes. Clasp clitoral cluster and maintain firm hold. Rotate by clasping perineal tissue.

HAND: As you support buttocks, straddling both cheeks, graze anal area with thumb.

Stage 5: Preorgasm

(three to five minutes)

TONGUE: Deepen gum or lip pressure against front commissure. Let her build friction. Focus tongue strokes more heavily on head, or maintain strong tongue-tip pressure against head.

FINGER: Maintain fingertip grasp of clitoral cluster. As you maintain contact with clitoral cluster in come-hither clasp, use thumb to stimulate frenulum.

HAND: Continue to provide support and stimulate anal area.

Stage 6: Orgasm

(less than one minute)

TONGUE: Focus on pressing your tongue into clitoral head. Use gums as strong point of resistance to her movements.

FINGER: As you feel orgasmic contraction, maintain fingertip pressure against clitoral cluster and frenulum.

HAND: Focus on maintaining position as she enters period of spasmodic orgasmic contractions. Use your hand to press up against buttocks and keep clitoral head aligned with tongue.

COMMENTS: In this routine, focus on the pressure you are increasing with your gums and fingertips. Focus on understanding the balance between pressure and tongue strokes.

ROUTINE 3

This routine will introduce more complex tongue strokes as well as further integrate the use of fingers. We will also introduce anal stimulation. This is a base line routine in that all major areas are now being fully stimulated.

▶ Level: Intermediate ◀

Stage 1: First Kiss
(less than one minute)

TONGUE: Nibble your way through the first kiss. Spend time nibbling inner lips before nibbling clitoral head.

FINGERS: Clasp perineal tissue throughout first kiss. Index finger should be inside, thumb on outside.

HAND: Support buttocks. Massage with fingertips.

Stage 2: Establishing Rhythm
(three to five minutes)

TONGUE: Alternate vertical, horizontal strokes. Introduce diagonal strokes.

FINGERS: Focus single finger on clitoral cluster. Massage the area behind frenulum with index finger as you press it from the outside with thumb.

HAND: Press thumb against perineum.

Stage 3: Developing Tension

(five to ten minutes)

TONGUE: Gum press. Introduce new tongue stroke: a literary lick, or rope-a-dope, in which you alternate flat, still tongue with attack of gentle strokes against head.

FINGERS: Insert second finger into vaginal entrance. Maintain fingertip clasp against clitoral cluster, but raise tops of fingers so you are pressing into clitoral cluster against vaginal ceiling. Continue to stimulate frenulum with thumb.

HAND: Maintain support and thumb-press against perineum.

Stage 4: Escalation

(three to five minutes)

TONGUE: Continue routine from previous stage, but increase gum pressure. Try scraping front commissure and top of head with teeth. Press teeth against clitoral area.

FINGERS: Maintain proper come-hither clasp of three key areas: frenulum, clitoral cluster.

HAND: As you support buttocks with your hand, straddling both cheeks, graze anal area with thumb.

Stage 5: Preorgasm

(three to five minutes)

TONGUE: Deepen gum pressure. Focus on strokes that are more varied and less predictable in rhythm. Introduce an element of dissonance into the process.

FINGERS: As you maintain position, massage clitoral cluster without breaking fingertip contact.

HAND: Insert tip of thumb into anus.

Stage 6: Orgasm

(less than one minute)

TONGUE: Maintain deep gum pressure. As you feel orgasmic contractions, apply light tongue flourishes that "spike" the orgasm.

FINGERS: As you feel orgasmic contraction, maintain pressure with fingertip against clitoral cluster and thumb tip against frenulum.

HAND: Focus on keeping legs together, supporting clitoral contact, and maintaining tip of thumb in anus. Observe contractions of sphincter in addition to pelvic floor muscles.

COMMENTS: In this routine, you are integrating all major components. In particular your fingers are stimulating the clitoral cluster and the frenulum with one hand, and the anus with the thumb of the other. You are also varying your tongue strokes and introducing a dash of unpredictability into the rhythm that teases and heightens the process. During orgasm, in addition to maintaining firm pressure throughout, you are also "spiking" the process with light tongue flourishes.

ROUTINE 4

This routine continues to build on the baseline techniques described in Routine 3. Changes to baseline are in bold text.

▶ *Level: Intermediate* ◀

Stage 1: First Kiss
(less than one minute)

TONGUE: Nibble your way through the first kiss. Spend time nibbling inner lips before nibbling clitoral head. Or return to long, slow lick.

FINGERS: Clasp perineal tissue throughout first kiss. Index finger should be inside, thumb on outside.

HAND: Support buttocks. Massage with fingertips.

Stage 2: Establishing Rhythm
(three to five minutes)

TONGUE: Alternate vertical, horizontal strokes. Introduce diagonal strokes.

FINGERS: Use index finger and thumb to clasp perineum: the perineal clasp.

HAND: Turn her over onto her side and spread legs as though she's doing a semisplit.

Stage 3: Developing Tension

(five to ten minutes)

TONGUE: With her on side and legs in semisplit position, focus on internal licks. Start inside with tongue against frenulum and work your tongue from inside out with strokes that start inside and then end on clitoral head.

FINGERS: Insert second finger and maintain strong perineal clasp.

HAND: As she maintains semisplit position on side, insert thumb tip into anus.

Stage 4: Escalation

(three to five minutes)

TONGUE: Return to standard position and gum-press. Try scraping front commissure and top of head with teeth. Press teeth against clitoral area.

FINGERS: Maintain proper come-hither clasp against frenulum and clitoral cluster.

HAND: As you support buttocks, straddling both cheeks, graze anal area with thumb.

Stage 5: Preorgasm

(three to five minutes)

TONGUE: Deepen gum pressure. Focus on strokes that are more varied and less predictable in rhythm. Introduce an element of spontaneity into the process.

FINGERS: Insert third finger, widen vaginal entrance. As you maintain position, massage clitoral cluster without breaking fingertip contact. Or use "under and up" technique to snake arm through leg and insert middle and fourth finger. Let her tap frenulum against index finger.

HAND: Insert tip of thumb into anus.

Stage 6: Orgasm

(less than one minute)

TONGUE: Maintain deep gum pressure. As you feel orgasmic contractions, apply light tongue flourishes that "spike" the orgasm.

FINGERS: As you feel orgasmic contraction, maintain fingertip pressure against clitoral cluster, as well as thumb-tip pressure against frenulum. Or if you are doing "under and up" position, increase the pressure of your index finger as you tap against frenulum.

HAND: Focus on keeping legs together, supporting clitoral contact, and maintaining tip of thumb in anus. Massage anus as she experiences orgasm and slowly remove during contractions.

COMMENTS: In this routine, we varied her position in the "developing tension" phase, which allowed us to lick the area of clitoral cluster. We returned to the baseline routine, but we inserted a third finger and also proposed an "under and up" alternative to the standard come-hither clasp; we also massaged the anal area as she experienced orgasm.

Advanced Routines

Once you have mastered the baseline routine of the intermediate phase, as well as the modifications of Routine 4, it's time to improvise, create your own routines, discover new techniques, and pursue innovative approaches that require a high degree of proficiency and awareness.

Routine 5: The Tease

This is an approach that focuses almost exclusively on tongue strokes and the stimulation of the visible parts of the clitoral network; in short, no finger work. Additionally, the tongue strokes employed on the surface of the vulva should be as light and gentle as possible. In this manner, you will *ever so slowly* tease her to orgasm, and when it comes, it will be sharp and light, without the fullness that results when internal parts of the clitoris are manually stimulated as well.

- During the process, do not insert a single finger inside her, and use your hands to vary her position and the angle of her vulva to your tongue.
- Push up her legs with both of your hands and prop her up on her butt, or raise a single leg; position her on her side in a semisplit position and use your tongue to graze the inside of her vaginal ceiling and clitoral cluster.
- But, in general, stick to the surface. Get as close to licking her as possible *without* actually licking her, and then graze the clitoral head.
- Use your thumbs to part her outer lips and fully reveal the clitoral head and hood, and then skim the area with your tongue.
- This approach will prove excruciatingly tantalizing. Intersperse your light tongue strokes with a still, flat tongue that she can move against, but don't provide her with the friction or resistance that would generally come as a result of applying your fingers and gum.
- Once she enters the preorgasm phase (and it may take a while), bring her legs together as close as possible, while still having access to her vulva, and place your hand under her butt.

- With your free hand, press up on her pubic mound and tighten her vaginal entrance. Continue to apply light strokes against the head until she comes.

Routine 6: The Tao of Cunnilingus

In general, Taoist sex practices are designed for genital intercourse and emphasize a few key principles: postponement of male gratification and the importance of female satisfaction; regulation and conservation of male ejaculation (you don't orgasm every time you have sex); and the understanding that an orgasm is not the same as ejaculation. This last point is more relevant to men in that it encourages recognizing when you're on the verge of orgasm and then pulling back. (When you hear someone talk about male "multiple orgasm" and "going all night" without cessation, this is generally what's meant—going to the verge repeatedly and pulling back as opposed to ejaculating repeatedly.)

Because women have a true capacity for multiple orgasms, the distinction between the preorgasm and orgasm phase as well as the emphasis on pulling back from the verge, is less important. However, you can heighten the experience of her orgasm by prolonging the period spent in the preorgasm phase (but make sure you are confident in your ability to bring her to orgasm in the first place before you focus on delaying the process). In the Tao of Cunnilingus, the man focuses on keeping the woman in the preorgasm phase as long as possible, getting her close to orgasmic contractions without triggering them.

- Prior to her entering the preorgasm phase, consider playing with some light restraint. Although it's by no means required, this element will definitely add some fun and excitement to the proceedings and is very much in keeping with the spirit of this routine.

- Once you recognize that she's entered the preorgasm phase and is on the verge of orgasmic contractions, reduce the pressure on her clitoris and slow down; cease your tongue strokes altogether.
- Remove your mouth completely from her vulva for three to five seconds and then return to applying firm pressure.
- You can maintain your come-hither clasp against her clitoral cluster, but reduce the pressure.
- After the pause of tongue strokes, bring her back to the verge of orgasm, and then once again reduce the pressure. Get her as close to orgasmic contractions as you can before pulling back. (In fact, you can even bring her to her first contraction, and then pull back. She won't lose the orgasm, but it may erupt from her when you return a few seconds later with your tongue strokes.)
- When you're ready to let her come, apply a deep firm gum-press and hard tongue strokes in combination with your come-hither clasp.
- Additionally, you can get in on the fun by bringing yourself close to orgasm by rubbing against her leg and then pulling back at the same time. (Note: This is also a great way of developing stamina and discipline if you suffer from premature ejaculation. By rubbing against her leg, you have more control of the process and can take yourself close to orgasm without actually ejaculating.)

Conclusion

THERE'S A POIGNANT SCENE in the film version of Milan Kundera's book *The Unbearable Lightness of Being*. Tomas and Tereza, a young married couple, are living in Prague at the start of the oppressive Soviet occupation of the 1960s. Tomas has always been an avid womanizer and, even in marriage, is unable to relinquish his erotic adventures with other women. He lives lightly and freely, but his marriage is shallow and empty. Tereza is imprisoned by the heaviness of her love for Tomas, tortured by his "lightness."

The couple takes advantage of an opportunity to emigrate to Geneva, thinking it might provide them with a fresh start, but Tomas, much to Tereza's disappointment, continues his life of ardent philandering. One day, unable to bear it any longer, Tereza impulsively leaves him and returns alone to doomed Prague.

Only after she's left does Tomas finally realize that his life is empty without Tereza; so he makes a difficult decision—to return to

Prague, where he'll live in perpetual poverty, never again to work as a surgeon, never again to know freedom of speech or liberty of choice. In short, he accepts the inherent heaviness of life.

We follow Tomas as he crosses the border into Czechoslovakia. We watch as he hands over his passport, permanently, to the border guard.

Back in Prague, Tomas returns to his old, dark, shabby apartment, where Tereza lies sleeping. She wakes up and can't believe her eyes. They embrace with tears in their eyes and that night they make love for the first time. Of course they've had sex countless times; but this is the first time they are truly making love; their bond to each other finally has a sacramental element, born of Tomas's sacrifice to be with her, consummated in the heaviness of their true love for each other.

As Kundera explains, the title, *The Unbearable Lightness of Being*, comes from a meditation on the philosophy of Nietzsche, who said that we should live every moment of our lives as though we were sentenced to repeat it over and over, forever and ever, for all eternity. We should live each moment as though we were creating an eternal, unchangeable work of art.

Easier said than done. We can't live every moment as though it were eternally indelible; it's simply too hard and would make life much too heavy. So instead we attempt to escape and live with a sense of lightness. We postpone our goals, we get into ruts, we distract ourselves with trivialities, but deep down we know that we could be living life more fully according to our potential; lightness is undermined by a sense of heaviness; hence, the unbearable lightness of being.

For all of his sexual adventures and numerous lovers, it takes Tomas years before he is finally able to make love. He is only able to do so by turning his back on the lightness of meaningless affairs and embracing the heaviness of a committed relationship.

We may not be able to live each moment as though we were going to repeat it over and over for all eternity, but we can make love that way; we can kiss our beloved knowing that we want that kiss, like a pebble cast into a still lake, to ripple and undulate for all eternity. Like Tomas returning to Tereza's embrace, we can make love totally and indelibly, with all the heaviness and substance of our being. As George Bernard Shaw wrote, "When you loved me I gave you the whole sun and stars to play with. I gave you eternity in a single moment, strength of the mountains in one clasp of your arms, and the volume of all the seas in one impulse of your soul."

When she comes first, she comes forever.

Appendices

1. Manual Stimulation During Foreplay

A suggested routine:

Position yourselves side by side, flat on your backs; drape your arm across her abdomen. This puts you in an ideal position to stimulate her dexterously with your fingers for prolonged periods of time, without tiring, as your arm is at rest and your wrist is supported by her pubic bone. This position also encourages you to focus on the right types of manual stimulation: gentle, rhythmic, external, as opposed to the wrong type—forceful, blunt, internal.

There are three basic steps to manual stimulation:

First, lying side by side—the base of your palm on her pubic mound, your fingers loosely draping her vulva—use a single finger (index or middle) to gently begin your exploration: trace the perimeters of her labia, both inner and outer; caress her inner thighs with your fingertips; stroke her vaginal entrance in a gentle come hither motion (actually the mirror image of this motion since your palm is facing downward), as though skimming the surface of a pond or softly petting a cat in the area right above its nose, between the eyes.

Then gently stimulate the peak of her clitoral head with a single soft fingertip in rhythmic circles.

Next, like you're petting the cat again, use short come-hither motions to approach the clitoral head from its underbelly (the area known as the frenulum), barely grazing her vaginal entrance.

Then, stimulating from the area just above the head where the outer labia meet—the front commissure—brush against the head in a downward motion with the soft surface of your fingernail and fingertip.

Now use two fingers to squeeze the head on either side.

Next, take those same two fingers, reach inside her vaginal entrance, press your fingertips against her vaginal ceiling, and grab hold of her pubic bone. In this position, your fingers are wrapped against the clitoral head. Massage the area just behind the head, where a cluster of sensitive nerve fibers intersect. As opposed to the light manual stimulation of the previous gestures, this position provides a more firm, still pressure. Depending

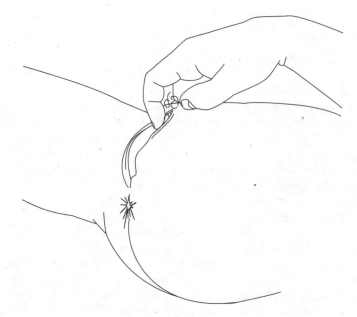

Manual Stimulation #1

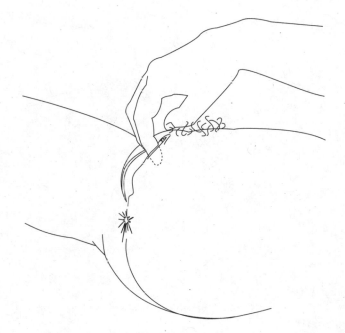

Manual Stimulation #2

on her level of arousal, you may well feel the clitoral cuff swell around the vaginal entrance and lightly clamp your fingers.

Consider inserting a third finger, as long as you work up to it.

Now, still in this position—whether with two or three fingers—make small, rapid movements from left to right, massaging both her clitoral cluster and head.

Now, remove your fingers and press the flat palm of your hand against her vulva, fully straddling its boundaries. Make your palm like a wall, and let her press into it—this stimulates the majority of nerve endings in the area of the vulva, especially those in the labia that often get neglected. Let her do the pressing. Often, in both manual and oral stimulation, men make the mistake of assuming that they need to take the lead and provide the majority of the stimulation—hence, all the fuss about tired tongues or worn-out wrists. If you ever feel this sort of fatigue, you're probably working hard but not necessarily well. More often than not, all you need to do is provide a consistent point of resistance and pressure, whether it's the tip of your tongue or the flat palm of your hand.

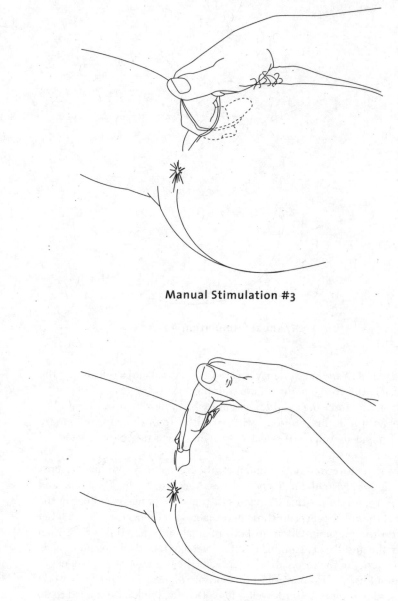

Manual Stimulation #3

Manual Stimulation #4

Lying next to her, alternate regularly between these three types of stimulation, and trust your instincts as to when to change position.

Or you might want to vary your approach and have her turn over on her stomach. Approach her from above, insert your thumb into her vaginal entrance, and use it to massage her clitoral cluster rhythmically while your index and middle fingers stimulate the head.

No matter what your approach, take your time and allow her gradually to build up the sexual tension that will ultimately be released through orgasm—perhaps sooner than later. When it comes to manual stimulation, it doesn't matter if you're a lumberjack or businessman—no matter what your trade, we all need strong "working hands."

2. Some Pointers on the Use of Restraint

Restraint, as proposed in this book, does not involve *any* pain or danger, but rather promotes trust and titillation.

Use soft restraints: neckties, scarves, or ribbons, or go out and purchase Velcro wrist and ankle bands that are created specifically for sex play.

Try restraining her hands separately (perhaps to bedposts, if you have them) or else together. If you're tying them together, do so above her head rather than behind her back (you don't want to cause discomfort or cut off her circulation).

In restraining her legs, don't make the mistake of separating them widely and tying them individually (the classic image being that of a woman's arms and legs stretched taut and tied spread-eagle to the four corners of the bed). Instead, tie her legs together at the ankles so that she can assume a number of body positions.

A Word of Caution

- In restraining anyone—be it man or woman—*never* tie any part of the person's neck.
- Do not cover her face, or do anything that might prevent her from breathing properly. Some people enjoy the experience of being tied and gagged, but the latter can easily be achieved in a way that does not prevent her from breathing (for example, tying a thin strip of cloth *around* her head and mouth rather than stuffing anything *in* her mouth).

- If she's truly helpless and cannot liberate herself on her own, never leave her alone, not even for a few moments.
- Do not restrain her for prolonged periods of time.
- Always respond to any aspect of the experience that makes her uncomfortable and adjust your behavior accordingly. Sometimes her protests can be part of the fantasy, so decide on a clear signal, like a word or sentence, for clearly interrupting the experience and bringing it to a halt.

3. Modifications of the Standard Position

If you grapple with sexual dysfunction:

There are two variations on the standard position that are enjoyable in their own right, but also serve as an aid to those men who suffer from sexual dysfunction, specifically premature ejaculation or erectile disorder.

In the case of the former, it should be noted that cunnilingus is an intensely erotic activity, and while it does not necessarily compel the "firing" of a hair trigger as intensely as genital penetration, it can certainly lead to premature ejaculation (PE), particularly as she approaches climax.

If you grapple with PE, have her lie toward the foot of the bed, legs dangling off and vulva aligned with the edge of the bed. Place a pillow on the floor and kneel down in front of her (she can also hang her legs over your shoulders). In this position, you are able to effectively provide a full range of oral techniques while simultaneously avoiding the type of physical contact and friction against your own body that might lead you to ejaculate.

As for erectile disorder, some men complain of not being able to stay aroused or of losing their erection during cunnilingus. If this is a problem, adopt the main position described at the start of this chapter, with a slight variation: instead of positioning yourself between her legs, try straddling one of her legs with your own and resting your penis against her leg.

You can even apply some massage oil and rub gently against her leg throughout your session. In this way, you remain connected to her body and should find yourself amply aroused. Additionally, see *penetration* in Chapter Twenty-one for a technique that intersperses genital thrusting with cunnilingus and may help you to maintain an erection.

4. The Protected Kiss, Part 1

In Chapter Eighteen, we talked about the importance of safe sex and latex. Now it's time to actually get out your gear and put it to good use. If you've already stimulated her manually during foreplay and are taking appropriate precautions, you know that you should be wearing latex gloves, perhaps ones that were bought specifically for the occasion from a sex-gear catalog. They can be purchased in various colors and textures—some are lightly powdered or lubricated—and feel less "medical" than the standard issue.

Now it's time for the dental dam. First off, make sure you've got an unused, clean one. (They're disposable and come by the dozen so this shouldn't be an issue.) Dams are also designed for anal play, so make sure that the one you're using for her vulva does not come into contact with her anal area, as the latter may contain bacteria that you don't want mingling with the former.

Tongue Tip: *When selecting a dental dam for cunnilingus, try the Glyde "LOLLYES" brand. It was designed specifically for oral sex and is the only barrier of this type to have been given FDA approval. According to the makers, LOLLYES stands for "Lips on Lickable Latex—YES!" Unlike traditional dental dams, Glyde barriers are ultra-thin, long, and transmit sensation extremely well. They come in various colors, and some are even scented. They can be ordered directly from sheerglydedams.com, or else from sex-gear catalogs such as blowfish.com. These ultrathin barriers are definitely worth the investment.*

Apply a few drops of water-based lubricant to her vulva (oil and latex don't mix well) and place the barrier against the entire area, covering the vaginal entrance. In using a dental dam, know that she will not be able to respond to the direct moistness of your tongue. Instead, she will respond to the transmission of vibration and sensation through the latex. Almost all of the tongue techniques in this book can be implemented through a latex barrier, but it may be necessary to adjust them slightly and focus on deeper, more intense versions, since very light actions may not transmit well.

- When using a dental dam, think of your tongue as an active force for applying pressure, and also integrate your gums and teeth into the action. In terms of the first kiss, you'll want to use the ice-cream lick described earlier, but when you reach her clitoral head, instead of brushing over it lightly with your tongue, softly press the flat surface of your front teeth against it.

When you are using a dental dam, it would be a bald-faced lie to say that your abilities as a cunnilinguist are not somewhat handicapped; they most certainly are, roughly by a factor of about 30 to 40 percent. It's hard to make up for the loss of a wet, unfettered tongue and the electrifying sensations that it can deliver with the gentlest of touch. But it's by no means impossible. You have to work within new limitations and compensate with creativity and perseverance. Know and accept your limitations at the outset, and you'll be able to make up for them in other gratifying ways.

Instead of thinking of the dental dam as a barrier to sensation, employ it as a new tool to enable pleasure:

- Brush her clitoral head with the edge of the dam.
- Or insert one end of the dam inside her vagina and press up against her clitoral cluster as you wrap the remaining piece up around the clitoral area. Use both hands to "polish" the clitoris like an exquisite pearl.

Question: When it comes to oral sex and dental dams, why even bother? Why not just stimulate her manually and go straight to genital penetration?

Answer: Because even with a dental dam, she can experience quite a bit of pleasure from oral sex, and there are things you can accomplish through the combination of your tongue, teeth, gums, and lips that you cannot achieve simply with your hands or penis. *The main barrier to pleasure when using a dental dam is not physical, it's mental.*

There's so much more to cunnilingus than simply the tongue: there's the rhythmic pressure that you can apply with your teeth, gums, and lips; there's the combination of oral and manual stimulation that you're in a position to lavish upon her in abundant supply; there's the focus and attention that you can pay to her process of sexual response; and finally there's the *complete* experience of the act—the physical, mental, and emotional sum total, which is so much greater than any of its individual parts. Just because one of your actors may be partially restrained doesn't mean you can't still put on one hell of a show.

5. The Protected Kiss, Part 2

Question: "I'm currently dating a few different women, so I guess you could say I'm not monogamous, at least not now. I'm at a point in my life where I just want to have fun, but that doesn't mean I don't want the fun to be safe, so I use a latex barrier when going down on a girl. The tricky part is keeping the barrier in place while trying to use my fingers inside her vagina. I wish I had four hands—two to keep the latex in place, and another two to finger her with. Any suggestions?" (Chad, 34)

Answer: The issue you raise regarding latex barriers, namely keeping them in place and not being able to use your fingers for manual stimulation, is probably the single greatest complaint that's leveled against them—that, and the reduced sensation that often accompanies their use.

Some folks have tried to devise fairly original ways for keeping the barrier in place. Such innovations include: using dental dams in combination with tight-fitting "crotchless" panties; wrapping small elastic garter straps around each thigh and then attaching them to the respective corners of the dental dam. I've even heard of people making panties out of Saran Wrap. I'm not going to go to the effort of describing these various "jerry-rigs" (use your imagination) because frankly I haven't heard any raves on their behalf and they just seem downright silly.

Sometimes it helps if she holds the dam in place while you apply tongue strokes, but probably the best solution is simply to get comfortable holding the barrier in place with one hand while using your free hand to manually stimulate her. I know that doesn't solve your problem, so I'm going to suggest that you approach the challenge in a new way: rather than focus on how to "free up" your hands, focus on how best to stimulate her clitoral cluster while using your hands to keep the barrier in place.

- Start with a dildo (a soft, plastic replica of the male penis that comes in various sizes and textures); buy one with a thick ta- pered head (at least a couple of inches in diameter) that will fit snugly inside her vaginal entrance.
- Insert the head of the dildo (the first couple of inches) into her vaginal entrance. It should fill her without being uncomfortable, and expand the area of her frenulum, as would happen during in- tercourse. Most important, the dildo should remain secure in- side her without requiring the assistance of your hands.
- Hold the dental dam in place and use your thumbs to massage her frenulum while you apply tongue strokes to the clitoral head.
- Apply delicate tongue strokes to the clitoral head; her clitoral cuff should tighten around the dildo, particularly if you've intro- duced it after building up substantial sexual tension.
- Or, using a standard-size vibrator, slowly insert it most of the way into her vaginal entrance. Only the base of the vibrator, and an inch or two of the shaft, should protrude. Set it to a low vibra- tion. You'll find that as you hold the dental dam in place, you should be able to push down on the base of the vibrator with your chin, or one of your wrists, and gently massage her.

Finally, if you and your partner(s) are serious about your cunnilingus (and also have a sense of humor), think about purchasing a device called "The Accommodator," otherwise known as a "chin-dong." The Accom- modator is a strap-on dildo that fits onto the end of your chin and is se- cured with elastic headbands (like a catcher's mask). When wearing a chin-dong, you literally look as though you have a penis growing out of your face, so get ready for some laughs. But a chin-dong does the trick in that you can easily manipulate it and apply tongue strokes at the same time.

6. The Scarlet Kiss

The truth is that you don't *have* to avoid oral sex just because she's menstruating, but you may be inclined to. In general, both men and women are sensitive to issues of taste, odor, and hygiene when it comes to cunnilingus, and these sensitivities are amplified when she's experiencing her period. But thanks to the invention of the simple tampon, you can give her flow-free, spine-tingling head 365 days a year (assuming she's game, of course; some women experience a marked decrease in sexual desire when they're menstruating, while others feel a substantial increase. It all depends upon her unique chemistry).

- Prior to foreplay, let her insert a fresh tampon and clean off the area of her vulva with a washcloth.

Now you're ready to go, and can implement most of the tongue techniques discussed in this book.

- As always, focus on gentle, light movements and the application of rhythmic, persistent pressure.
- It makes sense for the applicator string to be pulled down and generally out of the way, although sometimes the string can be used to great effect to caress and swipe the clitoral head in combination with your tongue.
- You'll want to hold off on the full use of your fingers, but that's okay since the tampon is actually their proxy. As you lead her through the process of arousal, her pelvic muscles and clitoral cuff will tighten around the tampon and help to stimulate the orgasm. The tampon will also apply pressure against her clitoral cluster.
- Just because you're not inserting your fingers doesn't mean you can't use them around her vaginal entrance, labia, perineum, and anal area. And if you want, you can tuck a finger in under the tampon, and help to press it against her clitoral cluster and clitoral cluster. Even with a single finger inside her, the experience will remain flow-free.

There's no reason why she shouldn't be able to experience an orgasm in this manner. In fact, the efficacy of this technique just goes to show that the female orgasm is largely produced through stimulation of the dense clitoral nerve endings that populate the surface of the vulva and are unobstructed by the tampon.

In terms of the Scarlet Kiss and your safe-sex routine, even if you're using latex, know that the likelihood of both transmitting and receiving an STD rises when she's menstruating, as viral bacteria, such as HIV, are more prevalent in her blood. So, even if you're using the tampon method in combination with a dental dam, you may want to consider avoiding cunnilingus altogether during her period if you are also engaging in the Protected Kiss.

7. The Virgin Kiss, His First Time

Question: "I really want to go down on my girlfriend, but I've never done it before and I'm a little nervous—not about smell or anything like that, but about doing it right and pleasing her. Any advice for a first-timer?" (Eric, 21)

Answer: Take note:

1. Make sure she's been amply aroused during foreplay.
2. Take your time.
3. Be as gentle and rhythmic as possible. Forget everything you've seen in porn films, but be confident. Don't confuse being gentle with being listless. Be strong of mind and tongue.
4. Focus on what you can see: her labia (inner and outer), the commissure and frenulum, her vaginal entrance, her perineum, and clitoral head; enjoy her entire vulva.
5. Don't make a rush for her glans (the clitoral head); it's extremely sensitive, so focus instead on other parts of the vulva at the outset.
6. Start with slow, broad strokes: up, down, left, right. Observe what works and what does not. Don't be afraid to ask her if something feels good, but don't hit on with a barrage of questions either.
7. Let her know how much you're enjoying it; tell her how good she tastes.
8. Keep it simple and rhythmic. Focus on the basic routines outlined in this book. Avoid the fancy stuff; don't worry about stimulating the clitoral cluster—for now.
9. Trust your instincts; relax into a meditative zone where you're not thinking so much as doing.
10. Take a pleasure-focused approach, not an orgasm-focused one. She may or may not come your first time out. But that doesn't mean she won't enjoy herself thoroughly.

8. The Virgin Kiss, Her First Time

Question: "My boyfriend wants to have oral sex with me, and I'm both excited and nervous: excited because it's my first time receiving it and I don't know what to expect, but also because I've never had an orgasm during intercourse. I'm able to orgasm when I masturbate, just not when I'm with a guy. I've faked it in the past, but I really like my current boyfriend, and we're talking about getting married, so I wanted to be up front and honest. He's very enthusiastic about oral sex and really believes that I'll be able to have an orgasm that way, but I just don't know. The truth is that I've never let a guy do that to me, go down, because I'm not completely comfortable with a guy seeing, tasting and smelling me. Any thoughts?" (Lynn, 23)

Answer: Your boyfriend is right. You do have a much better chance of experiencing an orgasm through cunnilingus than through genital intercourse. That's because the clitoris is the powerhouse of the orgasm, and is best stimulated through persistent, rhythmic pressure.

Genital intercourse generally doesn't provide the clitoris with the stimulation necessary to take you through the process of sexual response, which is why you're able to orgasm when you masturbate.

The fact that you are able to experience an orgasm via masturbation is an extremely positive sign—f you couldn't, you might very well not be able to come via cunnilingus either. Masturbation is the first step toward training your body and mind to work together in the production of pleasure. So you're definitely on the right track. You're "wired" to orgasm.

- The main thing is to relax and take a pleasure-oriented approach. Don't focus on your orgasm; focus on enjoying the experience. It's great that your boyfriend is enthusiastic about cunnilingus; just make sure that he takes a pleasure-oriented approach as well, and doesn't become fixated on your orgasm.
- Make sure you've engaged in ample foreplay and that you're stimulated and ready to go. Think about the types of manual stimulation that enable you to come via masturbation.
- If a vibrator or dildo is part of your routine, you might encourage your boyfriend to incorporate it into the act. You might even want to let him watch you masturbate, or better yet, try masturbating yourself with *his* hand.
- Don't be shy about letting him know what feels good and what doesn't—be sure to praise him when it feels good, and be constructive when it doesn't—when it comes to feedback in the area of sexual performance, the male ego bruises *easily.*

Since you've never had a guy perform oral sex on you, prepare yourself for a roller coaster of physical sensations: some will feel terrific; others might feel new and strange, overwhelming, or even uncomfortable. Let him know if you want him to change what he's doing. As sex columnist and author Anka Radakovich writes of her first time receiving cunnilingus, "I was breaking in the front seat of my new car and got so excited by the tingling sensation that I accidentally hit the gearshift and plowed right into the garage door, smashing the front end. Imagine explaining this one to the insurance adjuster."

As for your shyness about allowing him to see, smell, and taste you, you're not alone, and there are some easy steps you can take to help relax you:

- Incorporate a bath or shower into foreplay; light candles; let him massage you with scented oil. But also appreciate your boyfriend's eagerness and know that most men love the sight, taste, and smell of the vulva and get incredibly turned on when giving cunnilingus. Hopefully, your boyfriend's enthusiasm will prove contagious and you'll be able to ease into the experience.

- Relax, let go, and focus on your process of sexual response. Try to get into the same frame of mind as when you masturbate. Stay in touch with your body, focus on receiving pleasure, and feel your way through the process. Most women tend to fantasize much more during oral sex than they do during intercourse, so don't be afraid to let go and allow your imagination wander.

- Also know that it may take a few attempts before you're able to climax, so don't get frustrated. You may get *very* close, but still not come.

- Finally, if you feel that you are close to coming, but are unable to get yourself over the edge, consider masturbating yourself the final "few yards," especially since you know that you are able to come this way. We tend to think of masturbation as a private, sometimes even shameful, act, but the fact is that both men and women fantasize about watching their partners masturbate. Since you've already been open and honest enough with each other to talk freely about your inability to experience an orgasm during intercourse, you should be candid and comfortable enough in your relationship to understand the importance of masturbation. He'll most likely enjoy watching you stimulate yourself past the point of no return, *especially* since he helped get you 90 percent of the way there.

- If you're not open to masturbation, let him use his tongue to take you as far as you can get down the road of arousal, and try genital penetration in the female superior position—where you get on top and have a higher degree of control over the position of his penis, as well as the rhythm and pressure that's applied against your clitoris. A lot of women also feel more comfortable touching themselves during intercourse, so you can combine masturbation and penetration.

Above all, just try to enjoy the pleasure of cunnilingus. Even if you are unable to reach orgasm the first time around, rest assured you're on the path toward experiencing one.

9. The Pregnant Kiss

There's absolutely no reason not to enjoy cunnilingus during pregnancy, unless her doctor has specifically prohibited her from engaging in sexual activity, say in the case of a history of miscarriage, where uterine contractions can stimulate premature labor. Oxytocin—the chemical released during sexual activity—is also released during the uterine contractions of labor. In fact, synthetic oxytocin is sometimes used to induce labor, and a doctor may even recommend sex and orgasm as way of stimulating it.

In most cases, however, cunnilingus is an important way of maintaining a healthy sex life throughout all stages of pregnancy. In fact, she'll probably appreciate the attentions of your tongue all the more. According to *The Girlfriends' Guide to Pregnancy* by Vicki Iodine.

"The best news about the changes 'down below' is that many Girlfriends feel like they live in a state of constant sexual arousal because their organs are engorged with blood. My Girlfriend Tracy says that she became nearly orgasmic if she walked very far because the action of her legs rubbing together was like never-ending foreplay."

CAUTION: When pregnant women enter their second trimester, they are advised not to lie flat on their backs for prolonged periods of time, as this flat position could cut off the circulation of blood from the vena cava and affect the process of oxygenation within her body. Remedy this issue by placing a pillow underneath her hip and lower back (either side will do) and then tilting her slightly.

Another benefit of pregnancy is that she may be able to have orgasms much more easily, and they may be more intense and longer lasting. This is because her uterine contractions are stronger and more sensitive to the release of oxytocin during sex.

The flip side of all this arousal is that she may feel like she's in a constant state of sexual tension as her genitals are persistently engorged with blood. It's often during pregnancy that women first discover their potential for multiple orgasms by dint of sheer necessity.

Since cunnilingus is more up close and personal than any other sexual act, you might notice some changes during pregnancy: she might experience some spot-bleeding around the time she would normally menstruate. This light bleeding is nothing to worry about and should not be confused with the heavy bleeding that is usually symptomatic of an entopic pregnancy or impending miscarriage. Also, you might notice that her clitoris is engorged with blood, causing her labia to enlarge and change color—usually they become darker. Her natural lubrication could take on a thicker texture and more distinct odor. Be sensitive to these changes, know that she's probably sensitive to them as well, and find your comfort zone as a couple.

During pregnancy, the Three Assurances are more important than ever. Be sure to let her know that she smells great, tastes great, you find her beautiful in every aspect, and you genuinely enjoy going down on her.

10. Useful Toys

Question: "I'm fairly inexperienced in the art of cunnilingus, and I can't get my hands and tongue to work together—it's just too hard to concentrate on both at the same time. What can I do?" (Geoff, 32)

Answer: Try introducing a vibrator into your action. No matter what your skill level, a vibrator can prove to be a valuable addition to a cunnilingus session.

If your girlfriend doesn't already own a vibrator for masturbation, then buying one together can be fun and, perhaps, daunting: there's no shortage of sizes, shapes, textures, styles, and add-ons to choose from.

But as far as specifically choosing a vibrator that will augment your cunnilingus session, once again *form should follow function.* Many men make the mistake of thinking that the way to employ a vibrator is to thrust, jab, and penetrate, in cheap imitation of the penis during intercourse. This being the case, many vibrators are designed to resemble the male form.

Just as you focused your tongue and fingers on the application of gentle rhythmic motions that engage the visible aspects of the vulva, as well as the first couple of inches inside the vagina, use the vibrator in a similar fashion.

Think of the vibrator as a proxy for your tongue and fingers, not as the introduction of a plastic penis. Just because it resembles a penis doesn't mean that it should be used as one. To that end, a standard "wand-shaped" vibrator, four to six inches long, with the diameter of a quarter, will do just fine. You're mainly going to engage only the first couple of inches, so really length is immaterial.

Most vibrators are encased in a hard plastic shell, or else softened by a jellylike silicone sheath. Either type will do, but select a vibrator that is firm and solid, with just a bit of soft bend to it. In short, pick a no-frills toy that is reliable, unthreatening, comfortable, and easy to handle.

As with any tool, what matters most is how you use it. During a cunnilingus session, feel free to introduce the vibrator anytime after the first kiss, but know that it's best applied once you are well into your session and approaching the preorgasm phase.

While you can warm up and ease in by using the vibrator to gently stimulate all of the visible aspects of the vulva—labia, perineum, on and around the clitoral head—use it as a substitute for your fingers. Keep it set to a low speed—a diffused, persistent hum that gradually builds in resonance within her.

- Insert the vibrator into her vaginal entrance (use lubricant if necessary). Stay close to the entrance, and focus on her clitoral cluster. Gently thrust the vibrator in and out. Remember, since you're focusing on her vaginal entrance, the range of the motion should not exceed the first inch or two of her vaginal canal.
- Work primarily with the tip of the vibrator. Take your time; let the vibrator rest against her vaginal entrance; this slow, small movement should cause her clitoral cuff to tighten around the vibrator.

Tongue Tip: Once you've been stimulating her for a while, insert a finger or two underneath the vibrator and push up on it. This will enable the vibrator to really massage her clitoral cluster.

Xerox this blank template and use it to create your own routines

▶ **Stage 1: First Kiss** *(less than one minute)*

TONGUE: _____

FINGERS: _____

HAND: _____

▶ **Stage 2: Establishing Rhythm** *(three to five minutes)*

TONGUE: _____

FINGERS: _____

HAND: _____

▶ **Stage 3: Developing Tension** *(five to ten minutes)*

TONGUE: _____

FINGERS: _____

HAND: _____

▶ **Stage 4: Escalation** *(three to five minutes)*

TONGUE: _____

FINGERS: _____

HAND: _____

▶ **Stage 5: Pre-Orgasm** *(three to five minutes)*

TONGUE: _____

FINGERS: _____

HAND: _____

▶ **Stage 6: Orgasm** *(less than one minute)*

TONGUE: _____

FINGERS: _____

HAND: _____

BOOKS BY IAN KERNER, Ph.D.

SHE COMES FIRST
The Thinking Man's Guide to Pleasuring a Woman

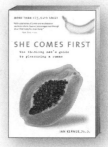

ISBN 978-0-06-053826-2 (paperback)
"Required reading for all men who are dating and all women who
are wondering why they're not satisfied."
—Cindy Chupack, Writer/Executive Producer of *Sex and the City*

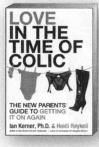

LOVE IN THE TIME OF COLIC
The New Parents' Guide to Getting It On Again

ISBN 978-0-06-146512-3 (paperback)
Funny and frank, *Love in the Time of Colic* will help parents take
the charge out of this once-taboo subject, and put it back where it
belongs—in the bedroom.

SEX RECHARGE
A Rejuvenation Plan for Couples and Singles

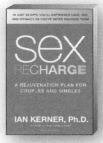

ISBN 978-0-06-123462-0 (paperback)
"Kerner makes intimacy intimate again, as well as downright
lustful. You'll walk away trusting your instincts instead of
subscribing to the fabricated ideas of what sexy 'should' be."
—Stephanie Klein, author of *Straight Up and Dirty*

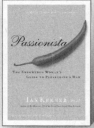

PASSIONISTA
The Empowered Woman's Guide to Pleasuring a Man

ISBN 978-0-06-083439-5 (paperback)
"*Passionista* satisfies the reader with tasty morsels of sexual
enlightenment, nibble by nibble, bite by bite."
—Lou Paget, bestselling author of *How to Be a Great Lover*

BE HONEST—YOU'RE NOT THAT INTO HIM EITHER
Raise Your Standards and Reach for the Love You Deserve

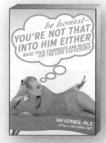

ISBN 978-0-06-083406-7 (paperback)
Kerner explores the battlefield of sex, hook-ups, go-nowhere
relationships, and the dismal dating treadmill, simultaneously
arming women with a sharper set of insights and the
tools for change.